T0225876

ANXIETY AND DEPRESSION IN PRIMARY CARE

This book provides practical information about depression and anxiety in primary care, with a focus on the approach in different countries and incorporating global ranges/prevalence, risk factors and health burdens, including those associated with COVID-19 and its pandemic.

To ensure the challenges of a wide international primary care community are reflected fully, authors from different world regions – Africa, Asia Pacific, East Mediterranean, Europe, Ibero-Americana-CIMF, North America and South Asia – have co-contributed to individual chapters on the detection and management of depression and anxiety in primary care in their own countries, including the screening tools used, how widely these tools are adopted and by whom and current policies. As well as the medical model, it also presents the alternative viewpoint that feeling low or anxious is part of the human condition and the attention should be on supporting people in their journey through life, struggling to deal with the mainly social challenges they meet, rather than defining these problems as disorders or diseases requiring identification and treatment.

Addressing primary care detection and management of mental health issues across the globe, the book will be an invaluable practical aid for family medicine practitioners and the wider primary and community care teams and a useful reference for those involved in policy setting at regional and national levels, including ministries of health.

WONCA Family Medicine

About the Series

The WONCA Family Medicine series is a collection of books written by worldwide experts and practitioners of family medicine in collaboration with The World Organization of Family Doctors (WONCA).

WONCA is a not-for-profit organization and was founded in 1972 by member organizations in 18 countries. It now has 118 Member Organizations in 131 countries and territories with membership of about 500,000 family doctors and more than 90 per cent of the world's population.

Family Medicine: The Classic Papers

Michael Kidd, Iona Heath, Amanda Howe

International Perspectives on Primary Care Research

Felicity Goodyear-Smith, Bob Mash

The Contribution of Family Medicine to Improving Health Systems: A Guidebook from the World Organization of Family Doctors

Michael Kidd

How To Do Primary Care Educational Research: A Practical Guide

Mehmet Akman, Valerie Wass, Felicity Goodyear-Smith

ICPC-3 International Classification of Primary Care

Kees van Boven and Huib Ten Napel

Family Medicine in the Undergraduate Curriculum: Preparing medical students to work in evolving health care systems

Valerie Wass and Victor Ng

Anxiety and Depression in Primary Care: International Perspectives

Sherina Mohd Sidik and Felicity Goodyear-Smith

For more information about this series please visit: https://www.crcpress.com/WONCA-Family-Medicine/book-series/WONCA

ANXIETY AND DEPRESSION IN PRIMARY CARE

International Perspectives

endorsed by the World Organization of Family Doctors (WONCA)

EDITED BY

Sherina Mohd Sidik, MBBS, MMED (Fam Med), PhD (Community Health)
Universiti Putra, Malaysia, Malaysia
Member of the WONCA Working Party on Research

Felicity Goodyear-Smith, MBChB, MGP, MD, FRNZCGP (Dist)
The University of Auckland, Auckland, New Zealand
WONCA Chair Working Party on Research

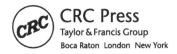
CRC Press
Taylor & Francis Group
Boca Raton London New York

CRC Press is an imprint of the
Taylor & Francis Group, an **informa** business

Designed cover image: Shutterstock – image number - 1859547085

First edition published 2024
by CRC Press
2385 NW Executive Center Drive, Suite 320, Boca Raton FL 33431

and by CRC Press
4 Park Square, Milton Park, Abingdon, Oxon, OX14 4RN

CRC Press is an imprint of Taylor & Francis Group, LLC

© 2024 selection and editorial matter, Sherina Mohd Sidik and Felicity Goodyear-Smith; individual chapters, the contributors

ISBN: 978-1-032-48940-7 (hbk)
ISBN: 978-1-032-47951-4 (pbk)
ISBN: 978-1-003-39153-1 (ebk)

DOI: 10.1201/9781003391531

Typeset in Minion Pro
by KnowledgeWorks Global Ltd.

Contents

Foreword by Karen Flegg

"*Anxiety and Depression in Primary Care*" is a much needed publication from the World Organization of Family Doctors (WONCA) Working Party on Research.

The editors, Sherina Mohd Sidik (Malaysia) and Felicity Goodyear-Smith (New Zealand), have brought together a diverse range of authors from 25 different countries to contribute their knowledge on this important topic to health professionals in primary health care and to their interested patients.

The book aims to provides practical information about depression and anxiety in primary care. It will meet the needs of an international audience from a large variety of country situations and addresses situations in high, middle and low income countries. The 34 chapters ensure a comprehensive coverage of the topic.

One of the important messages of the book is that while there is a call for an increase in the global diagnosis and management of depression and anxiety, some also express concerns that people feel distress and experience existential angst as part of a natural human condition, and there is a need to not to over-medicalise normal emotional responses.

As early as Chapter 1, Dawit Wondimagegn points out the magnitude of the issues under discussion: "Mental illness in the world accounts for the greatest global burden of disease (13%), and the largest percentage (28%) of the non-communicable burden of disease."

From each of the seven WONCA regions of the world namely, Africa, Asia Pacific, Europe, Ibero-America, North America and South Asia, several local authors present the situation in their own country. This provides a most interesting collection of 20 case histories outlining country situations. One cannot help but make comparisons but must also notice the many similarities and the universally significant burden of depression and anxiety. The vulnerable populations of migrants, refugees and war zone populations are also covered.

The remaining chapters cover approached, assessment, interventions and improving practice. The editors sum up with reflections on the normal changes in mood versus changes that constitute disorders which may require active intervention. The role of family doctors as the trusted carers deciding a balance between treatment and waiting, medication and other interventions support services is presented

This book will contribute to improving consideration of depression and anxiety throughout the world. This is turn will no doubt improve health outcomes and better achieve "Health for All".

Associate Professor Karen M Flegg
The Australian National University Rural Clinical School
WONCA President
MBBS(Hons), MIntPH, FRACGP, FACRRM, GradDipClinEpi
Rural Clinical School
School of Medicine and Psychology
The Australian National University
Canberra, Australia

Preface

According to the World Health Organization (WHO), approximately 280 million people in the world were living with depression and 301 million with anxiety disorder in 2019.[1,2] A systematic review published in *The Lancet* estimated an additional 53.2 million cases of major depressive disorder and 76.2 million cases of anxiety disorder globally in 2020 due to the COVID-19 pandemic, an increase of 27.6% and 25.6%, respectively.[3] The WHO's Comprehensive Mental Health Action Plan 2013–2030 calls for increased mental health services and strategies for promotion and prevention of these mental health conditions in all countries, with an emphasis on non-specialised health care providers in community settings.

Experiencing stress is part of daily living, a natural response which prompts us to address challenges and threats we encounter. When we feel overwhelmed by the stresses in our lives and feel unable to cope, we experience distress. Feeling distressed at times is also part of the human condition. People respond differently, and not everyone may perceive a specific situation as a threat. You will see in this book that opinions differ as to when it is considered that existential angst becomes a diagnostic condition of depression or anxiety requiring formal intervention.

Most people with mental health issues are likely to initially present in community settings. Physical and mental health are inter-related, and both need to be addressed in primary care to improve health outcomes. This is regardless of whether depression or anxiety is formally diagnosed or whether the general practitioner recognises a change in mood due to stress, and works with a patient to help improve their lifestyle choices, health and wellbeing.

This book provides an international perspective on how depression and anxiety are identified, diagnosed and managed in primary care. It will appeal to a global audience of clinicians, academics and policy makers involved in the detection and management of mental health issues in the community. It will be of interest to medical practitioners (general practitioners, family physicians, family medicine specialists, community psychiatrists, public health and other primary care doctors), family practice, school and other primary care nurses and other primary care providers such as medical assistants, paramedics, social workers and school counsellors, community pharmacists, psychologists, psychotherapists, occupational therapists and counsellors, medical and nursing students – anyone involved in mental health care in the community, as well as the interested lay public. We hope you enjoy this book and find it useful in your practice.

Sherina Mohd Sidik
Felicity Goodyear-Smith

REFERENCES

1. Institute of Health Metrics and Evaluation. Global Health Data Exchange 2023 [cited 2023 May]. Available from: https://vizhub.healthdata.org/gbd-results/.
2. World Health Organization. Mental disorders Geneva 2022. Available from: https://www.who.int/news-room/fact-sheets/detail/mental-disorders (accessed May 2023).
3. Santomauro DF, Mantilla Herrera AM, Shadid J, et al. Global prevalence and burden of depressive and anxiety disorders in 204 countries and territories in 2020 due to the COVID-19 pandemic. *Lancet*. 2021;398(10312):1700–12.

Editors

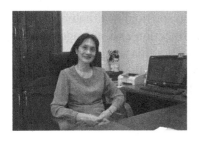

Sherina Mohd Sidik, MBBS, MMED (Fam Med), PhD (Community Health), is a family medicine specialist and professor in family medicine at Universiti Putra, Malaysia. She has published over 150 peer-reviewed papers as well as 7 books and 20 book chapters. She is a member of the WONCA Working Party on Research, the Primary Health Care Research Consortium (PHCRC) Advisory Committee and the SHIFT-MH International Strategic Advisory Board (ISAB), Institute of Mental Health, University of Nottingham, United Kingdom.

She has a special interest in community mental health and serves on several national committees on mental health in primary care and community settings. She has conducted and participated in many studies on mental health in Malaysia, which include studies on the detection of depression and anxiety in the community, primary and secondary care, schools, institutions of higher learning and high-risk populations such as adolescents, women, the elderly, patients with chronic diseases and cancer and carers. Her current research focuses on interventional studies to improve the quality of lives of patients suffering from depression and anxiety in these populations.

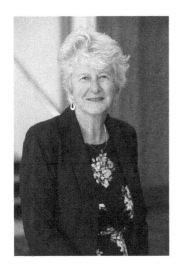

Felicity Goodyear-Smith, MBChB, MGP, MD, FRNZCGP (Dist), is a general practitioner and professor of general practice and primary health care at the University of Auckland, Auckland, New Zealand. She has a long involvement with WONCA, including being the past Chair of its Working Party on Research. She has previously co-edited three books in the WONCA Family Medicine series: *How to Do Primary Care Educational Research* (2021), *How to Do Primary Care Research* (2018) and *International Perspectives in Primary Care Research* (2016), and has also contributed chapters to three other books in this series. Dr Goodyear-Smith was the founding editor-in-chief of the *Journal of Primary Health Care* and has been co-editing it since 2022. She has published over 340 peer-reviewed papers as well as a number of books and book chapters.

She has always seen that a core feature of family medicine is the trusted relationship between clinician and patient. Family medicine provides holistic care, addressing the physical, mental, social and spiritual health and wellbeing of patients and their families. Initial identification and management of depression and anxiety sits in primary care, whether this is supporting people to deal with the challenges of stressful situations in their lives or formally diagnosing a mental disorder, as this book explores.

Contributors

Noor Ani Ahmad, MBBS, MPH
Director
  Institute of Public Health
  Ministry of Health
  Shah Alam, Malaysia

Mehmet Akman, MD, MPH, FP
Professor and Family Doctor
  Department of Family Medicine
  Marmara University
  Istanbul, Türkiye

Raquel Gómez Bravo, MD, MSc, PhD
Visiting Researcher and General
  Practitioner
  Department of Behavioural and
    Cognitive Sciences
  Faculty of Humanities, Education
    and Social Sciences
  University of Luxembourg
  Esch-Sur-Alzette, Luxembourg

Alice Einloft Brunnet, Bpsy, MSc, PhD
Assistant Professor
  Clipsyd Research Laboratory
  Paris-Nanterre University
  Nanterre, France

Richard Byng, MBBCh, MRCGP, MPH, PhD
Professor and Family Doctor
  Peninsula Medical School
  University of Plymouth
  Plymouth, England

Lidia Caballero, MD
Doctor
  Ministry of Public Health of
    Misiones
  Posadas, Argentina

Asma Chaabouni, MD, MSc (Psych Mental Health)
Family Doctor
  Faculty of Medicine of Tunis
  Tunis, Tunisia

Malek Chaabouni, MD, MRes
Assistant Physician
  Department of Pulmonology and
    Thoracic Oncology
  Asklepios Klinik Altona
  Hamburg, Germany

Julie Yun Chen, MD, CCFP, FCFP
Associate Professor of Teaching
  Department of Family Medicine
    and Primary Care
  The University of Hong Kong
  Hong Kong SAR, China

Weng Yee Chin, MBBS, FRACGP
Assistant Professor and Family
  Doctor
  Department of Family Medicine
    and Primary Care
  The University of Hong Kong
  Hong Kong

Saliha Serap Cifcili, MD
Professor of Family Medicine
  Marmara University School of
    Medicine
  Department of Family Medicine
  Istanbul, Türkiye

Aysegul Cömert, MD
Family Doctor
  Department of Family
    Medicine
  Ankara University School of
    Medicine
  Ankara, Türkiye

Lisa Cosgrove, PhD
Professor
  Department of Counseling and
    School Psychology
  University of Massachusetts
  Boston, Massachusetts

Yolanda Dávila, Psi, PhD
Professor
  Universidad del Azuay
  Cuenca, Ecuador

**Vinicius Jobim Fischer, Bpsy,
  MSc, PhD**
Psychologist
  Neuropsychiatric Hospital
    Center – CHNP
  Ettelbruck, Luxembourg

**Karen Flegg, MBBS, MIntPH,
  FRACGP, FACRRM,
  GradDipClinEpi**
Associate Professor
  Rural Clinical School
  Australian National University
    College of Health and
    Medicine
  Canberra, Australia

**Alison Flehr, BSc (Hons),
  GradDipPsych, PhD**
Research Officer
  Department of General Practice
    and Primary Care
  University of Melbourne
  Melbourne, Australia

**Felicity Goodyear-Smith, MBChB,
  MGP, MD, FRNZCGP (Dist),
  FFLM**
Professor and General Practitioner
  Department of General Practice
    & Primary Health Care
  University of Auckland
  Auckland, New Zealand

**Jane Gunn, MBBS, PhD, FRACGP,
  FAHMS**
Professor and General Practitioner
  Faculty of Medicine, Dentistry
    and Health Sciences
  University of Melbourne
  Melbourne, Australia

Pramendra Prasad Gupta, MD
Associate Professor
  Department of General Practice
    and Emergency Medicine
  BP Koirala Institute of Health
    Sciences
  Dharan, Nepal

**Lesca Cherise Hadley, MD, MBA,
  FAAFP, AGSF**
Associate Professor and Family
  Physician
  Department of Family Medicine,
    Texas
  Christian University Burnett
    School of Medicine
  University of North Texas Health
    Science Center
  Ft Worthssse, Texas

Amanda Howe, MD, Med, DCH, DRCO
Emeritus Professor and General
  Practitioner
Primary Care, Norwich Medical
  School
University of East Anglia
Norwich, England

Nurashikin Ibrahim, MBBS, MPH
Public Health Physician
Disease Control Division
Ministry of Health Malaysia
Putrajaya, Malaysia

Adelson Jantsch, MD, MPH, PhD
Family Doctor
Universidade do Estado do Rio de
  Janeiro
Rio de Janeiro, Brazil

Caroline Johnson, MBBS, FRACGP, GCUT, PhD
Associate Professor
Department of General
  Practice
University of Melbourne
Melbourne, Australia

Catherine Kaylor-Hughes, AFHEA, BSc (Hons), DPhil
Senior Research Fellow in Mental
  Health
Department of General Practice
  and Primary Care
University of Melbourne
Melbourne, Australia

Henry J. Lawson, MBChB, FWACP, FCGP
Senior Lecturer and Consultant
  Family Physician
Head, Family Medicine Unit
Department of Community Health
University of Ghana Medical
  School
Accra, Ghana

Christos Lionis, MD, PhD, FRCGP (Hon), FWONCA, FESC
Professor
School of Medicine
University of Crete
Crete, Greece

Vanessa Lomas-Marais, MBChB, MMed
Senior Lecturer and Specialist
  Family Physician
Department of Family and
  Emergency Medicine
Helderberg Hospital
Stellenbosch University
Tygerberg, South Africa

Diana López, MD
Lecturer
Universidad del Azuay
Cuenca, Ecuador

Bob Mash, MBChB, DRCOG, DCH, FRCGP (UK), FCFP (SA), PhD
Executive Head and Distinguished
  Professor
Department of Family and
  Emergency Medicine
Stellenbosch University
Tygerberg, South Africa

Sherina Mohd Sidik, MBBS, MMED (Family Medicine), PhD (Comm Health)
Professor
Department of Psychiatry
Faculty of Medicine & Health Sciences
Universiti Putra Malaysia
Selangor, Malaysia

Nagwa Nashat Hegazy, MSc, MD, DHPE, FAIMER
Professor and Family Doctor
Family Medicine Department, Faculty of Medicine
Menoufia University
Shebin El Kom, Egypt

Alan Ng Cheng Hin, MBChB, DipObst, DCH, DTM&H, MRCGP, CCFP, FCFP, MMEd
Assistant Professor
Department of Family Medicine
University of Ottawa
Ottawa, Canada

Amy Pui Pui Ng, BSc, MD, CCFP
Clinical Assistant Professor
Department of Family Medicine and Primary Care
The University of Hong Kong
Hong Kong SAR, China

Tijani Idris Ahmad Oseni, MBBS, FMCFM
Lecturer and Consultant Family Physician
Lifestyle and Behavioural Medicine Unit, Department of Family Medicine
Ambrose Alli University
Ekpoma, Nigeria

David Ponka, MD, CCFP(EM), FCFP, MSc (Int Primary Care)
Professor and Director Besrour Centre for Global Family Medicine
Department of Family Medicine
University of Ottawa
Ottawa, Canada

Silvia Reina, PhD, BSc
National Scientific and Technical Research
Council CONICET (Consejo Nacional de Investigaciones Cientificas y Tecnicas)
Universidad Catolica de las Misiones
Posadas, Argentina

Saniya Sabzwari, MBBS, MD, MHPE, Fellow ABFM
Professor Family Medicine
Department of Family Medicine
Aga Khan University Hospital
Sindh, Pakistan

Susan Senstad, BDed, MA(Clin Psych)
Writer and Editorial Consultant
Oslo, Norway

Allen F. Shaughnessy, PharmD, MMedEd
Professor
Department of Family Medicine
Tufts University School of Medicine
Boston, USA

Thomas Shima, DO, MS, FACOFP
Clinical Assistant Professor and
  Family Physician
Department of Family Medicine,
  University of Texas Southwestern
  Medical School
Dallas, Texas

Anna Stavdal, MD
Associate Professor and Family
  Medicine Specialist
Department of General Practice
University of Oslo
Oslo, Norway

**Victoria Tkachenko, MD, PhD, Dr
  Sci in Med (Gen Pract/Fam Med)**
Professor and General Practitioner
  Department of Family Medicine
  Shupyk National Healthcare,
    University of Ukraine
  Kyiv, Ukraine

Matías Tonnelier, MD
Family Doctor
  Vista Alegre Primary Care Center
  Neuquén, Argentina

Sabah Tuzun, MD
Associate Professor
  Marmara University Pendik
    Training and Research
    Hospital
  Department of Family Medicine
  Istanbul, Türkiye

**Pemra Cöbek Ünalan, MD, MSc
  (Cancer Biology and Genetics)**
Professor
  School of Medicine,
    Department of Family
    Medicine
  Marmara University
  Istanbul, Türkiye

Mehmet Ungan, MD
Professor and Family Doctor
  Department of Family
    Medicine
  Ankara University School of
    Medicine
  Ankara, Türkiye

**Miriann Mora Verdugo, MMed,
  PhD**
Professor
  Universidad del Azuay
  Cuenca, Ecuador

Dawit Wondimagegn, MD
Associate Professor and Consultant
  Psychiatrist
  Department of Psychiatry
  Addis Ababa University
  Addis Ababa, Ethiopia

CHAPTER 1

Global perspective on depression and anxiety

Dawit Wondimagegn

GLOBAL PREVALENCE AND RISK FACTORS

To contextualise mental health disorders, according to the World Health Organization (WHO), mental health is defined as "a state of well-being in which the individual realises his or her own abilities, can cope with the normal stresses of life, can work productively and fruitfully, and is able to make a contribution to his or her community".[1]

Mental illness in the world accounts for the greatest global burden of disease (13%), and the largest percentage (28%) of the non-communicable burden of disease.[2] A third of the years lived with disability are attributable to mental illness in adults worldwide.[3]

Severe mental illness (SMI) is generally understood to describe a cluster of disorders: schizophrenia, bipolar disorder and severe depression.[4] These disorders are often what people bring to mind when they think of mental illness. The people affected are seriously distressed, and their ability to take care of themselves is extremely impaired. They often live with a different sense of reality, can be quite disorganised in their thinking and management can be difficult. Unfortunately, they seldom come to primary care for help. Despite the obvious suffering of the individual, their family and the community, SMI affects only 0.8–6.8% of people worldwide.[5]

Much more prevalent are common mental disorders (CMDs) – depression, anxiety and medically unexplained symptoms, which represent the largest category of mental disorders. At any one time, 9.8–19.1% of people in the world are affected by CMDs.[5] CMDs cause significant individual, family and social suffering, often with serious financial implications due to impaired

DOI: 10.1201/9781003391531-1

work ability. Unlike the impact of SMI, most people with CMDs have appropriate hygiene and are organised and so do not draw attention to themselves. It may be difficult to know they are suffering unless they are asked about their symptoms and function.[6]

Our focus on CMDs is due to their high prevalence and frequent co-occurrence with other health issues. Screening patients who attend primary care and providing mental health treatment for those who need it is a cost-effective, non-stigmatising way of reducing mental suffering and improving the general health of a significant number of patients in primary care and surrounding communities.[7]

CMDs are more than simply feeling unhappy or fed up for a few days. Life stressors often become overwhelming because of insufficient social support and underlying psychological or biological vulnerability. We all go through spells of feeling sad, demoralised or unhappy, but when these feelings persist for weeks or months, it is probably a CMD.

How can someone tell if they are depressed? Depression affects people in different ways and can cause a wide variety of symptoms, ranging from lasting feelings of sadness and hopelessness, to losing interest in the things previously enjoyed and feeling very tearful. People with depression may have physical symptoms, such as feeling constantly tired; sleeping badly; having no appetite or sex drive; and complaining of various aches and pains, numbness or tingling. Depression is just one of the presentations of CMD.[8]

Anxiety is closely related to fear, or anticipating disaster, irritability and worry, with difficulty calming thoughts down. The patient may feel a sense of dread that something awful will happen, or feel haunted by past events that were terrifying. Like depression, anxiety shares many of the same physical symptoms such as restlessness, feeling jittery, having trouble concentrating and difficulty sleeping. Panic attacks are another manifestation of anxiety not uncommon in CMDs.[9] Often a patient will complain of only the physical symptoms, which may have been investigated with no physical cause found. Medically unexplained symptoms (MUSs) are a common presentation for CMDs, and treatment can help resolve the patient's symptoms and reduce their frequent visits to primary care centres.[10]

CMDs cause psychological suffering and interfere with family, social and occupational functioning.[11] The more severe the CMD, the more the functioning of a person is affected. At its most severe, CMDs can make a person feel suicidal, that life is no longer worth living. Sometimes CMDs can come on gradually. Many people continue to try to cope with their symptoms, often attributing them to physical causes, not realising how distressed they have become. It may take a friend or family member to suggest something is wrong. Generally, if symptoms are present most days for more than a month, professional help is needed. Many people wait a long time before seeking help, but it is best not to delay – the sooner help is sought, the sooner the patient will recover.[12]

There are no physical tests for CMDs, although the health provider may do a physical examination or blood tests to rule out other conditions that have similar symptoms, for example, thyroid disorder. Health care workers screen for CMDs by asking lots of questions. Patients should try to be as open as possible with their primary care worker (PCW) to determine if a CMD exists and how severe it is.[13]

Discussions between patients and PCWs or counsellors are confidential, although the worker can talk to a colleague or a specialist about the patient if it is for the patient's benefit. Breaking confidentiality to other appropriate people is necessary if there is significant risk of harm to either the patient or to others, or if informing a family member or mental health specialist would reduce that risk.[14]

The people in our lives can be our greatest source of comfort, but sometimes they are a significant cause of stress.[15] However, not every potential stressor is a risk to mental health for everyone. Another way of thinking about this is that distress does not usually lead to mental illness – no matter how distressed a person is, once the stressor has gone or has been adapted to (for instance, the death of someone important), their distress begins to fade.[16] But for some people, distress does not end once the stressor has gone, and they are at risk of developing a CMD.

Each person has a unique set of psychological resources, understanding of the world and way of perceiving things – what seems like a threat to one person may be experienced as an interesting challenge to another. The right amount of stress is valuable to us; it stimulates us to grow, develop and do better. However, it is important to match stressors in life with sufficient resources to deal optimally with the stress that is experienced. The more stress, the more support anyone needs.

Some experiences act as risk factors for CMD, although risk varies from person to person. Some things tend to stress and cause distress in most people – lack of work, job demands like long hours and poor pay, a sick child, school stress, health fears, financial concerns. These undermine personal needs for security and raise concern for family survival, which can lead to marital conflict and relationship stress.[17]

There is an important interaction between medical and psychological health – someone with a physical health problem is at greater risk of a CMD; similarly, a person with a CMD is at greater risk of a physical health problem. For example, a person with HIV is more vulnerable to a CMD. Having both HIV and a CMD can make it more difficult to take medications properly – the patient may forget, may not feel like making the effort or feel that the medications will not work so there is little point in taking them, worsening their HIV status.[18] In addition, having a CMD might make a person more vulnerable to HIV because they are less careful or feel more desperate with respect to sex. Or a mother who develops a CMD after giving birth may not find the energy and determination to ensure her baby is vaccinated or has access to clean water. This can cause the baby to be sick or even die, which worsens the woman's CMD.

A good family life while growing up contributes significantly to a person's resilience to withstand later hardships.[19] However, there are many difficult life experiences that can contribute to CMDs. Serious risk factors for the development of depression and anxiety include:

1. Domestic violence is often under-reported by those experiencing it and under-detected by health care providers. Domestic violence by one adult member of the household towards another can include physical, sexual and emotional violence. Domestic violence is associated with poor health, depression and suicide.[20]
2. Alcohol misuse becomes a problem when a person drinks to excess, it can cause or worsen CMDs and physical illness; lead to family violence, poor work and social function; and exacerbates disputes and arguments. It is associated with a higher risk of serious physical accidents. Overuse of alcohol can become a disorder of addiction when the individual's life revolves around alcohol, adversely affecting work, family and the community.[21]
3. Major life events like death and bereavement can be a risk for CMDs.[22]
4. Life role transitions can be a risk for CMDs.[23] For some patients, failing to complete culturally directed rituals relevant to life transitions worsen their mental distress, e.g., births and losses.
5. Disputes/arguments in the context of one's social relationships can be a risk for CMDs.[24]
6. Stigma and discrimination towards mental illness and the mentally challenged lead to an increased risk of CMDs and create a barrier to accessing health services and achieving occupational and social goals.[25]
7. Physical health disorders, especially chronic disorders such as HIV/AIDS, stroke or diabetes, make a person significantly more vulnerable to CMD.[26]
8. Physical and emotional violence and/or neglect and sexual abuse, particularly in childhood, are risk factors for later physical disorders and mental health distress and disorders. This is important in times of unrest and war as well. Screening for these risks will equip the PCW to be able to address the suffering of patients.[27]

WHO INITIATIVE ON UNIVERSAL COVERAGE FOR MENTAL HEALTH

The WHO initiative for universal coverage for mental health was launched for the years 2019–2023 with the vision for all people to achieve the highest standard of mental health and well-being. The initiative's target was to make mental health care accessible for 100 million more people in 12 priority countries. The WHO committed to employing two strategic actions focusing on advancing mental health policy, advocacy and human rights and scaling up interventions and services across community-based, general health and specialist settings to deliver the target by 2023. This initiative is believed to contribute towards the realisation of specific sustainable development goals.[28]

WHY MENTAL HEALTH SERVICES NEED TO BE INTEGRATED INTO PRIMARY CARE

"There is no health without mental health".[26] The link between mental and physical health is inextricable, whether you have a baby and become depressed, develop a chronic medical condition like tuberculosis (TB) or have a motor vehicle accident, and so on. We all want both our physical and mental health to be attended to by capable, well-trained people. Changing health care systems to ensure mental health services are available to all people through community primary care health clinics is an ambitious undertaking. Changing the current (most) mental health system from a centralised specialist service delivery structure to a tiered care approach involving PCWs in primary care centres, mid-level mental health professionals, psychiatrists and, importantly, traditional and religious healers in communities is complex.[29]

Because CMDs are so common, good basic mental health services are particularly needed in primary health care settings to ensure those suffering from mental health problems have adequate access to help and treatment.[30] Mental health integration in primary care health systems incorporates essential mental health services so that PCWs are confidently able to recognise and treat CMDs, which may or may not be concurrent with other medical issues. Important to note – this does not mean PCWs will see more patients, but rather PCWs will screen their patients for CMDs and treat those who are positive. In addition, with a tiered system of care, patients do not have to wait to be seen by mental health specialists. PCWs trained to deliver mental health services can help these patients, with support from mid-level mental health workers, such as master-level clinical psychologists, who might be periodically on site at primary care centres. As well, specialists could then be available for referrals, consultation on complex cases, in-patient treatment and ongoing professional assistance, as needed. Provision of early identification and treatment for patients with CMD in primary care is not only cost-effective, it reduces stigma and discrimination.[31]

Importantly, many patients in the global south see a traditional healer for both physical and mental health issues, and this is frequently sufficient for recovery. In implementing a tiered response to mental health, from primary care to specialist care, it is essential to not overlook traditional healers who are experienced in addressing culturally specific psycho-social-spiritual needs of people in distress.

Affiliations between traditional healers and contemporary health services benefit patients greatly.[32] Rather than assuming contemporary mental health methods developed in the West are intrinsically more effective and beneficial than traditional healing, an integrated approach to mental health care and training should actively encourage building relationships between traditional healers and local primary care personnel to create a positive environment for exchanging ideas and sharing best practices.[33]

WHAT HAPPENS WHEN DEPRESSION AND ANXIETY ARE NOT TREATED

When screening a patient for a CMD, it is important to look for issues that can cause or worsen CMDs and that represent threats to the safety of the patient, such as domestic violence, alcohol misuse and suicide risk.[34] CMDs (depression, anxiety and MUSs) are not trivial and not signs of weakness or something a sufferer can snap out of by pulling themselves together. The good news is that with the right treatment and support, most people can make a full recovery.

Mild CMD has some impact on daily life and might resolve with encouragement to resume or continue usual activities and maintain contact with friends, family and neighbours for support while working towards understanding the precipitating event. Talking through feelings can be helpful, whether with a friend or relative or spiritual advisor.

Moderate CMD has a significant impact on daily life, and psychotherapy is helpful when a CMD is not improving. Research has repeatedly shown that for mild to moderate CMD, psychotherapy is more helpful than antidepressants. There are psychotherapeutic modalities that can be delivered successfully at primary care settings.

Severe CMD makes it impossible to get through daily life and is often associated with psychotic symptoms. When it is this serious, it is no longer classified as a CMD, but as an SMI, requiring admission to hospital. Antidepressant, antipsychotic medications and other treatment modalities for mental health could be employed.

HOW DEPRESSION AND ANXIETY MAY MANIFEST IN DIFFERENT COUNTRIES AND CULTURES

As medical knowledge has grown over the centuries, physical disorders are better understood by medical science, with both treatment and prevention aligned accordingly. However, throughout history, mental distress, disorders and problems have also been attributed to non-scientific causes, such as punishment from God or demonic possession states. Although we now know a lot more about mental disorders, especially CMDs, their recognition and treatment remain rooted in the psychological, social and cultural circumstances of the person affected.[35]

CMDs are caused or worsened by social factors that determine both mental and physical health. For example, people who can be at risk of a CMD include parents when their child is chronically ill and they do not have enough money for medicine, someone diagnosed with HIV who cannot tell their family, someone who could never please their father and now has a boss that is unkind and rude or a woman who is raped and is too afraid to disclose this.

Despite distress and difficulties, a CMD patient can recover with a thoughtful combination of medical, psychological, social and spiritual assistance. Improved communication with the public about CMDs can promote respect for culturally accepted knowledge and beliefs about causes, initiate self-help and promote integration of contemporary mental health professional assistance when needed.

A CMD frequently presents as various medically unexplained physical symptoms. MUSs, also known as persistent physical symptoms or somatic symptoms, are commonly associated with psychological distress. MUSs can be traced to clear stressors in the patient's life, although the patient may not be aware of this association. Physical symptoms can be plentiful, but despite numerous patient examinations, these are found not to be associated with an underlying medical condition.

If five or more physical symptoms are documented with no underlying physical cause and with an accompanying decrease in function, the patient probably has MUSs. Sometimes a patient has a chronic medical condition that may in part explain their physical symptoms. Treatment can help decrease/relieve their physical symptoms by reducing their psychological distress, mitigating the patient's restless search for medical tests.

Why do many patients experience psychological distress with physical symptoms? Perhaps this is because we all tend to take physical symptoms more seriously. We know people can become ill and die if they do not attend to their bodily complaints. As well, there is no real separation between mental distress and the physical experience of it; we lose sleep, cannot eat, feel restless or exhausted – these are all physical symptoms that may be physical manifestations of mental distress. Experiences such as falling in love or grieving the death of a loved one can be accompanied by these physical experiences. Some physical symptoms commonly flag mental, not physical, distress, for example, particular types of headaches, burning all over, general numbness or bodily pain. The key to identifying CMDs is to link the onset or worsening of symptoms to the patient's stressors, even if the patient does not make or even rejects the link themselves.

Often people with CMDs attribute their depression, anxiety or MUSs to life's hardship and look to God to help them recover. This attribution and help-seeking is wise and in-line with recovery. Sometimes Western-trained mental health workers assume that telling the patient he or she has a mental illness will help the patient. This is not usually true, and may inadvertently contribute to the hardship of mental distress by stigmatising the person. Being told that one's mental distress is a "mental illness" may burden the patient further, with worry that they have a disease in addition to their problems and distress. Diagnosis of a mental illness may also introduce self-stigma as a sense of shame, self-blame, an assumption they will go mad and never recover; that they will be locked up indefinitely; or a feeling that God is punishing them.

We all must think carefully about psycho-education and mental health literacy and what we might be conveying, despite our best intentions. Stigma leads to discrimination, which reduces access to health care, education, employment, marriage, productivity and well-being. Families are also affected by stigma, which sometimes leads to a lack of support for their family member. For mental health professionals, stigma can mean they are viewed as abnormal, corrupt or evil, and psychiatric treatments are viewed with suspicion and fear.

Other groups are subjected to multiple types of stigma and discrimination at the same time, such as people with an intellectual disability, with a mental illness or who are also from a cultural or ethnic minority. The stigma of mental illness is worsened when combined with other stigmas, such as HIV/AIDS, ethnic or religious minorities or severe poverty.

Discrimination towards a mentally ill person can negatively affect medical treatment. For example, someone who is depressed or psychotic and breaks their leg may not receive good treatment because health workers are uncomfortable treating them. The mentally ill patient may not come forward for treatment of their physical illness or may be unable to follow up on taking medications or further appointments. This particularly applies to the severely mentally ill.

In conclusion, CMDs are common and treatable. They present a significant burden to individuals, family and society at large. Despite the availability of appropriate interventions, the detection, diagnosis and treatment of CMDs in primary care is limited. This could be due to several factors that include the individual patient presentations, the PCW's capacity to detect and the lack of resources to implement mental health policy that seek to integrate mental health into primary care despite evidence of effective interventions. A lot of advocacy for the implementation of mental health policies and programmes at all levels is required to improve the detection, diagnosis and treatment of CMDs in primary care all over the globe.

REFERENCES

1. World Health Organization. Promoting mental health: concepts, emerging evidence, practice (Summary Report). Geneva: World Health Organization; 2004.
2. World Health Organization. The global burden of disease: 2004 update. Geneva: World Health Organization; 2008.
3. Whiteford HA, Degenhardt L, Rehm J, Baxter AJ, Ferrari AJ, Erskine HE, Charlson FJ, Norman RE, Flaxman AD, Johns N, Burstein R. Global Burden of Disease attributable to mental and substance use disorders: findings from the Global Burden of Disease Study 2010. Lancet. 2013;382(9904):1575–86.
4. Gottesman II, Laursen TM, Bertelsen A, Mortensen PB. Severe mental disorders in offspring with 2 psychiatrically ill parents. Arch Gen Psychiatry. 2010;67(3):252–7.
5. Kessler RC, Aguilar-Gaxiola S, Alonso J, Chatterji S, Lee S, Ormel J, Üstün TB, Wang PS. The global burden of mental disorders: an update from the WHO World Mental Health (WMH) Surveys. Epidemiol Psichiatr Soc. 2009;18(1):23–33.
6. Kessler D, Heath I, Lloyd K, Lewis G, Gray DP. Cross sectional study of symptom attribution and recognition of depression and anxiety in primary care. BMJ. 1999;318:436–9. doi: 10.1136/bmj.318.7181.436
7. Crowley RA, Kirschner N; Health and Public Policy Committee of the American College of Physicians. The integration of care for mental health, substance abuse, and other behavioral health conditions into primary care: executive summary of an American College of Physicians position paper. Ann Intern Med. 2015;163:298–299. [Epub 18 August 2015]. doi: 10.7326/M15-0510
8. Goldberg DP, Huxley P. Common mental disorders: a bio-social model. Tavistock/Routledge; 1992.
9. Andrew G, Cohen A, Salgaonkar S, et al. The explanatory models of depression and anxiety in primary care: a qualitative study from India. BMC Res Notes. 2012;5:499. https://doi.org/10.1186/1756-0500-5-499
10. Khan MM. Medically unexplained symptoms. Pak J Neurol Sci. 2007;2(3):iv–vi.
11. Chopra P. Mental health and the workplace: issues for developing countries. Int J Ment Health Syst. 2009;3:4. https://doi.org/10.1186/1752-4458-3-4
12. Wang PS, Berglund PA, Olfson M, Kessler RC. Delays in initial treatment contact after first onset of a mental disorder. Health Serv Res. 2004;39(2):393–415. doi: 10.1111/j.1475-6773.2004.00234.x
13. Ali G-C, Ryan G, De Silva MJ. Validated screening tools for common mental disorders in low and middle income countries: a systematic review. PLoS ONE. 2016;11(6):e0156939. https://doi.org/10.1371/journal.pone.0156939
14. Blightman K, Griffiths S, Danbury C. Patient confidentiality: when can a breach be justified? Cont Edu Anaesth Crit Care Pain Med. 2014;14(2):52–56. https://doi.org/10.1093/bjaceaccp/mkt032
15. Harandi TF, Taghinasab MM, Nayeri TD. The correlation of social support with mental health: a meta-analysis. Electron Physician. 2017;9(9):5212–22. doi: 10.19082/5212
16. Schneiderman N, Ironson G, Siegel SD. Stress and health: psychological, behavioral, and biological determinants. Annu Rev Clin Psychol. 2005;1:607–28. doi: 10.1146/annurev.clinpsy.1.102803.144141
17. Harvey SB, Modini M, Joyce S, et al. Can work make you mentally ill? A systematic meta-review of work-related risk factors for common mental health problems. Occup Environ Med. 2017;74:301–10.
18. Unützer J, Schoenbaum M, Druss BG, Katon WJ. Transforming mental health care at the interface with general medicine: report for the presidents commission. Psychiatr Serv. 2006;57(1):37–47.

19. Masten AS, Best KM, Garmezy N. Resilience and development: contributions from the study of children who overcome adversity. Dev Psychopathol. 1990;2(4):425–44.
20. Gibbs A, Dunkle K, Jewkes R. Emotional and economic intimate partner violence as key drivers of depression and suicidal ideation: a cross-sectional study among young women in informal settlements in South Africa. PloS ONE. 2018;16;13(4):e0194885.
21. Gururaj G, Girish N, Isaac MK. Mental, neurological and substance abuse disorders: strategies towards a systems approach. Burden of Disease in India. 2005;226.
22. Utz RL, Caserta M, Lund D. Grief, depressive symptoms, and physical health among recently bereaved spouses. Gerontologist. 2012;52(4):460–71.
23. Mostert F. The role impairment associated with common mental disorders among first-year university students in South Africa. Master Thesis. Stellenbosch University. 2021.
24. Cyranowski JM. Practice considerations for behavioral therapies for depression and anxiety in midlife women. Menopause. 2022;29(2):236–8.
25. Maulik PK, Devarapalli S, Kallakuri S, Tripathi AP, Koschorke M, Thornicroft G. Longitudinal assessment of an anti-stigma campaign related to common mental disorders in rural India. Br J Psychiatry. 2019;214(2):90–5.
26. Prince M, Patel V, Saxena S, Maj M, Maselko J, Phillips MR, Rahman A. No health without mental health. Lancet. 2007;370(9590):859–77.
27. Arnow BA. Relationships between childhood maltreatment, adult health and psychiatric outcomes, and medical utilization. J Clin Psychiatry. 2004;65:10–5.
28. World Health Organization. The WHO special initiative for mental health (2019-2023): universal health coverage for mental health. World Health Organization; 2019.
29. Jenkins R, Othieno C, Okeyo S, Aruwa J, Kingora J, Jenkins B. Health system challenges to integration of mental health delivery in primary care in Kenya-perspectives of primary care health workers. BMC Health Serv Res. 2013;13(1):1–8.
30. Ivbijaro G, Funk M. No mental health without primary care. Ment Health Fam Med. 2008;5(3):127.
31. Ormel J, VonKorff M. Reducing common mental disorder prevalence in populations. JAMA Psychiatry. 2021;78(4):359–60.
32. World Health Organization. General guidelines for methodologies on research and evaluation of traditional medicine. World Health Organization; 2000.
33. Sullivan M. The new subjective medicine: taking the patient's point of view on health care and health. Soc Sci Med. 2003;56(7):1595–604.
34. Henriksen CA, Stein MB, Afifi TO, Enns MW, Lix LM, Sareen J. Identifying factors that predict longitudinal outcomes of untreated common mental disorders. Psychiatr Serv. 2015;66(2):163–70.
35. Kirmayer LJ. Cultural variations in the response to psychiatric disorders and emotional distress. Soc Sci Med. 1989;29(3):327–39.

CHAPTER 2

Alternative approaches to the 'diagnose and treat' model of care

Richard Byng

INTRODUCTION

Struggling with feeling low or anxious is part of the human condition. While we have developed evidence to help us understand how to address the problems of distress which people around the world struggle with, this chapter will challenge the dominant view that it is best to think about these problems as disorders or diseases like entities which need detecting and treating. I propose instead, following the tradition of others,[1] that we should focus both on individuals and their journey through life struggling to deal with the mainly social challenges they meet and also consider whole populations within localities. Common mental health problems are ubiquitous and present in every community and are more common in areas where social difficulties are more common – whether through war or other forms of violence, following unexpected losses or where activities that should bring a reward such as productive work are harder to engage in.

I consider the challenges of deciding how to act when what we call common mental health problems emerge from a complex mix of genetic disposition, prior trauma, the everyday losses of life and social adversity and that the internal psychological experiences individuals face fluctuate over time in ways which are not easy to predict. I touch on the implications of taking a systems approach in which, for example, alcohol use, low mood or depression and interpersonal partner violence are linked causally in different ways according to each situation, but for which there may be patterns. For example,

DOI: 10.1201/9781003391531-2

a man may start to drink more because of difficulties with working conditions and past trauma and start regularly beating his wife in front of his children when drunk. This is highly likely to lead to his previously well wife struggling with low mood and anxiety and also predispose his children to later violence, depression, heart disease and multiple other social and medical conditions.

Everything leads to everything, but how do we step back and think about what specific things we can do to address common mental health problems for the individual and the community? It is likely that solutions are similar in high-income countries (HICs) and in low- and middle-income countries (LMICs) and that lessons can be learned from each other. I believe that exporting some of the faulty ways of thinking and suboptimal solutions that have been developed over the last 50 years is not the right way forward. I will make a particular critique of how we think about common mental health problems and the diagnostic model, as well as how we portray the evidence of potential solutions – whether psychopharmacological, psychological or social. Working out what should be done in the diverse communities and health care systems of the LMICs might involve rethinking common beliefs about common mental health problems and also how we think about the populations we work with and systems we work in.

A CRITIQUE OF DIAGNOSIS

I start my critique by considering the nature of common mental health problems. What are they? How are they caused? And how should we think about them? On the face of it, it is quite simple. We can all identify with the idea of being sad or not enjoying things, the two core symptoms of what is called depressive disorder. If these persist and stop us getting on with life, then it's not unreasonable to consider that there is a problem. What has happened, however, is that symptoms have been turned into diagnostic entities, so that people are considered either disordered or not in a binary way. This is done by identifying clusters of symptoms (technically syndromes) and labelling them as disorders – perhaps because it sounds more medical and treatable than a syndrome. This is the 'nosological' approach to diagnosis, which in psychiatry only considers conscious symptoms and sometimes observable behaviours or appearances in the diagnostic process.[2] The 'lumping' of very different states together is a further problem, for example, depression can involve too much sleep or too little, agitation or being slowed down and over-eating or under-eating – clearly different physiological states. Furthermore, similar to many pain syndromes, and distinct from most of medicine where investigations are key to diagnosis, there is no objective assessment of underlying brain function in individual clinical practice.[3] It is also possible to be diagnosed with depression or anxiety with no understanding of what is causing it, not from any dysfunction of the brain nor from past traumas, losses or ongoing social stressors.

The last 50 years or more have been accompanied by considerable scientific efforts to understand which parts of the brain are responsible for this thing we call depressive disorder – how genetic predispositions have led to it and what kind of neurotransmitters are involved. This search has not been very fruitful, and the much publicised serotonin theory for depression has now been debunked.[4] In contrast, social inquiry has shown consistent effects first of major life events such as losing one's mother early in life[5] and, more recently, through a whole range of traumas or adverse childhood events which lead via complex mechanisms to a range of mental and physical health problems.[6,7] What is increasingly understood is that not only do most life stressors, traumas and losses lead to most mental health problems, i.e., different diagnoses, but also that there are common genetic predispositions – gene markers initially heralded as specific to one diagnosis are now shown to be linked to many, but with small effects for each.[8]

The ability to make a diagnosis based on a shorter list of eight questions helpfully formatted in questionnaires, such as the HAD and PHQ-9 and GAD-7, meant that general health workers, including family doctors and other practitioners, could be trained relatively easily to better 'detect' the common mental health diagnoses. Following the Defeat Depression Campaign of the 1990s, when new generations of antidepressants became generally available, much was written about how each doctor should diagnose every patient who passed through the primary care setting and met the criteria of depression.[9] Some doctors were less proficient than others, and screening programmes were developed so that patients could be identified by answering questionnaires, and if they scored positively then be seen by a health care practitioner for a possible diagnosis. This caused some confusion, as practitioners and patients did not understand the high level of false positives following screening, and scores on questionnaires effectively became diagnoses. Research aiming to show the benefits of this screening approach, however, failed to show any average improvement for those in family doctors' offices screened for depression.[10]

Anxiety disorder as a diagnosis was generally out of favour during the 1990s, perhaps as a result of the understanding that benzodiazepines used to treat individuals with anxiety over the previous 20 years had resulted in huge harm – or perhaps because depression was the common mental health problem which was seen as treatable. The diagnosis of anxiety has become more popular, however, particularly with the development of psychological therapy treatments, including in the United Kingdom (UK) the system-wide development known as Improving Access to Psychological Therapy (IAPT), or perhaps also because antidepressants started to be used for anxiety.

This focus on diagnosis as the first step in the management of mental health problems in family practice arguably led to a decreased emphasis on engagement, trust building and the therapeutic relationship which had been developed as an idea through practitioners such as Balint. It also probably reduced the emphasis on understanding the cause of distress, although general practitioners (GPs) continued probably through humanist instinct to be sensitive about social problems as causes for distress, inquiring about these when given the cue to do so by patients.[11]

Despite these conceptual and empirical weaknesses, diagnoses are no longer the domain of psychiatrists and other doctors and psychologists. In most HICs, anxiety and depression are recognised by the majority of the population as illnesses to detect, along with bipolar disorder and borderline personality disorder. Many individuals like the idea of getting a diagnosis (or other people being diagnosed) – some people feel it helps them understand what is happening to them, others that they are not alone and some now need a diagnosis to access various resources such as housing or income support. There is also evidence, however, that a diagnosis can reduce personal agency and the ability to make decisions about life.[12]

Some practitioners and patient groups have taken a different view. Perhaps most significantly to address problems of heterogeneity (people in the same diagnostic group having very different symptoms) and comorbidity, the US National Institute of Mental Health (NIMH) now encourages non-diagnosis-based research, focusing on underlying brain-based pathway dysfunctions.[13] While this arguably does not address social causes, it is perhaps a step in the right direction as it addresses the problem, introduced by the *Diagnostic and Statistical Manual of Mental Disorders, Third Edition* (DSM3), of classification according to symptoms, not causes.[14] The HiTOP project similarly avoids a purely diagnosis-based approach and looks at the range of symptoms across diagnoses.[15]

Many psychologists have long objected to diagnosis, preferring a formulation which takes account of family issues, relationships, social stressors and an understanding of psychological mechanisms which can be both beneficial and harmful. Practitioners also at times reject the diagnostic model. Family doctors appear to ignore it in everyday practice[11] while formally supporting the diagnostic model. The Critical Psychiatry movement in the UK is careful to avoid seeing itself as anti-psychiatry, like its predecessors in the 1970s, and is committed to a scientific understanding of the biological, psychological and social origins. However, unlike most national psychiatric professional bodies, it opposes diagnosis being the main vehicle for understanding mental health problems, with person-centred formulation just as an adjunct.[16]

Whereas in the 1980s Sartorius and others focused their efforts on psychosis,[17] interest in common mental health problems in LMICs has increased, and the mhGAP programme exemplifies the World Health Organization (WHO)–inspired mission to ensure all patients with depression and anxiety receive effective treatment.[18]

TREATMENT OF COMMON MENTAL HEALTH PROBLEMS

The analysis earlier, critiquing how we think about common mental health problems, goes to the heart of the problems with treatment. By making diagnosis the fulcrum of decision-making, we detract attention from the complexity of the human condition. The 'diagnose and treat' model could theoretically result in overall benefit to the population if we had effective treatment. In other parts of medicine, treatments have developed apace, with examples of 'great medicine' in the areas of orthopaedic surgery for hip and knee replacements, infectious diseases treatment (HIV and hepatitis C) and precision treatment of some cardiovascular events and some cancers (e.g., childhood leukaemia). In contrast, the effect sizes for common mental health problems such as depression or anxiety are small; the number needed to treat is about seven to nine to achieve one success in selective serotonin reuptake inhibitor (SSRI) treatment of depression.[19,20] We also know that mental health interventions have side effects, and so it is likely that there will be some benefit in the short term whilst others may be harmed. In the case of antidepressants, we are now increasingly seeing long-term harms through significant side effects following withdrawal of medication.[21]

In HICs, the number of antidepressant prescriptions has doubled every 10 years, and in some coastal cities in the UK, one in two adults has received antidepressants in any one year,[22] with co-prescribing of multiple medications for pain and distress now the norm.[23] Our focus has shifted to supporting people to come off medication, and rarely do we see calls to ensure that GPs have identified every case. Instead, our clinics are full of people ready to admit to mental health problems in the quest for treatment. Arguably, we have therefore been successful in reducing self-stigma, but along the way have failed to warn that treatments are not very effective and that we have very little way of knowing who is likely to benefit. An analysis of the Star-D data set illustrates the problem. Even with this exemplary care according to guidelines, remarkably few individuals who continued on antidepressants were found to have a positive outcome.[24]

Psychological therapy also suffers from the problem of similarly small effect sizes, with many therapeutic interventions showing no or very small effect, and only a few having moderate effect, some slightly higher than antidepressants.[25] The rise in the provision of cognitive behavioural therapy (CBT) in the UK has been a great achievement in terms of delivery success, but unfortunately, because of the low average effect size, it too is unable to provide a credible response to the large numbers of individuals coming forward and being diagnosed with depression or anxiety.

Increasingly, attention is being paid to the social causes of mental distress, but the number of high-quality trials is low, and the rapid expansion in the UK of social prescribing – the idea that practitioners can identify current social adversity or potential positive opportunities which could address distress – has also been an impressive delivery success. Unfortunately, there are few trials to prove that social prescribing is effective for low mood, and it seems unlikely, on the basis of non-randomised studies, that, as a treatment process, it will be any more effective than psychological therapy.

These small effects are likely to be related to an intrinsic difficulty in overcoming distress and other related symptoms (perhaps analogous to how difficult it is to treat leprosy or overcome obesity compared to the relative ease of treating lobar pneumonia). It is also likely, however, to be exacerbated by the misguided attempt at using diagnosis as the best means of understanding individuals' distress. Research on treatment based on diagnosis misses all the heterogeneity within such categories. Unfortunately, most treatments have been tested on individuals categorised as having depressive or anxiety disorders. This does not just relate to antidepressants, where expecting drugs to act similarly on individuals with too much or too little sleep, eating or activity makes little sense, but is also relevant for psychological therapies, so that an intervention designed to support someone whose thinking is said to be too concrete is unlikely to be helpful for someone who does not have that problem.[26]

There is the possibility that in the future we will be able to understand more about what is happening in somebody's brain, their neurotransmitter make-up and the operation of individual brain circuits and use personalised, individualised psychotropic care. But we are a long way from that. Social interventions seem less prone to having this problem, but are also harder to research. For example, it can be very difficult to recruit individuals burdened by debt in order to test whether debt relief will make a difference to their anxiety or depression.[27]

POPULATION AND SYSTEMS APPROACHES

The Alma Ata agreement of 1978[28] described a visionary future of primary care and affords a framework to bring together individuals' and communities resources with those of statutory services to provide individual care across health and other sectors. Population-based approaches come in a range of guises. While we have seen how mental health problems are not very treatable with medication, it seems likely that, because of their nature, they are likely to be improved (even if unpredictably) by a small degree by multiple interventions or broader self-help opportunities. Much of the resource for this will be within the individual, their family and community, as well as through physical assets such as lakes, hills or parks.

Goldberg and Huxley developed the model of 'pathways to care', illustrating that of those seeking help, only some are diagnosed in primary care, and some are passed on to secondary care.[29] This model has helped those designing systems in both HICs and LMICs to consider how to ensure those with the most significant mental health problems gain specialist care. However, it does not fully recognise individuals nor the important role of families and community assets. It also does not address the inequalities of access we have seen in most settings since the inverse care law was first described.[30] These linear systems with pathways into more intensive care appear to have been accompanied by a range of clinical 'cultural' phenomena. Firstly, the idea that as practitioners, we are responsible for treating individuals – a need to 'fix them'. This seemingly positive idea can lead to problems when the treatments are not very effective. In contrast, an opposite response to the 'demand' we have created is to say depression is 'not a problem for medicine' and individuals need to 'sort things out for themselves'. The combination can lead to confusion, hopelessness or anger. Such 'clinical cultural' ideas held by practitioners might be driven by fear. Fear of disappointing patients or fear of being accused of negligence provides an impetus to treat. This risk aversion can contribute to systems with long waiting times and dissatisfied patients and workforce.

Related cultural phenomena are found in professional organisations, as well as voluntary sector campaign groups which may gain from promoting the idea that we need to diagnose and treat more people. The media further contribute by talking up new fixes and rarely publicising the low effect sizes of medications or neutral trial results.

WAYS FORWARD

Addressing these problems will not always be easy. Finding solutions might require looking across our systems, understanding patient flows, population needs and our clinical and community cultures. Here we explore options at both clinical and population levels. There are positive examples across each continent and techniques such as asset-based community development[31] alongside the values articulated at Alma Ata.[28] Countries where psychiatric systems are less developed may have advantages, both because systems and pathways have not been set in stone and because there may be less of a culture within the population believing that mental health problems are similar to other diseases.

For primary care practitioners in everyday practice, some specific changes can build on current strengths. Primary care practitioners are skilled at engaging individuals and supporting them to feel that they can be helped. In the UK, the DESTRESS project has reshaped the consultation model based on what a lot of experienced practitioners do already and on what patients want.[32] It is being developed further into an approach with three lenses: Strength-based, trauma-informed and diagnosis-aligned. The first step is to build engagement and trust, the second step is to understand rather than diagnose and the third is to develop a shared plan together. Rather than launch in with a list of questions to obtain a diagnosis of anxiety or depression, practitioners are encouraged to do what many do anyway, which is listen to their patients; understand what is troubling them, including any social problems; and, with consent, enquiring about what past losses and traumas have led to their difficulties.

As part of building this shared understanding, a more medical or psychological approach might be helpful, with questions from the standard psychiatric history-taking used to understand the nature of what is happening in the brain, rather than just for coming to a diagnosis. For example, questions about mood can help identify individuals who feel low and slowed down for long periods or whether within a day there is rapid variation between anger and agitation and irritability, whether feelings of hopelessness are linked to self-harm and whether any episodes of elation last hours or weeks. Questions about thinking patterns can help develop a shared understanding about whether an individual has a tendency to paranoia and believing people are trying to harm them or whether they rarely think about others and dwell on negative thoughts about themselves. Questions about perception can be used both to ensure psychosis (e.g., hallucinations) is not missed and to identify symptoms of dissociation (e.g., the world not feeling real) and flashbacks of past trauma. Answers to these traditional psychiatric questions can therefore be used to develop the shared understanding so it includes links between what is happening in the social and psychological worlds. This can help individuals identify which social factors might be changeable in their lives. Diagnosis can be part of this formulation, but does not have to be, as often patients find that a good shared understanding means that a diagnosis is less likely to be requested.

There are positive signs that similar ideas are being developed across the world. In Burma, a randomised controlled trial (RCT)[33] has shown that transdiagnostic community-based mental health treatment for comorbid disorders can have a positive impact on mental well-being. In Uganda an RCT of group-based interpersonal psychotherapy for low mood has shown positive outcomes[34] and has been scaled up to be delivered to 130,000 individuals in Zambia and Uganda.[35] This approach combines individual work with the spread of ideas within the community through group-based work and spread beyond those attending groups.

Practitioners may also take on the role of supporting communities and populations in understanding their local situation in order to tailor support as well as engage in prevention. In Zambia a common element treatment approach working with couples has been shown to reduce intimate partner violence and alcohol use in an RCT.[36] This shows how the role of primary care practitioners in health care teams can work with local mental health teams and other voluntary sector organisations. Interestingly this is the vision now being developed in the UK with the Community Mental Health Framework.[37] This policy initiative diminishes the importance of the diagnostic model by emphasising individuals' strengths, collaboration across organisations and social support for individuals such as debt relief or better relationships. Rather than the Pathways to Care model,[29] networks of opportunities of social and psychological support are promoted. Evaluating such initiatives is complex and requires a systems approach rather than RCTs. The development of these approaches also requires political willpower with practitioner leaders and local managers working together to shift prevailing psychiatric models towards whole-person, whole-system ways of working. In the UK there is an emerging belief that this can be part of the answer to our problem of over-medication and long waiting lists for specialist mental health therapy and a population which increasingly identifies itself as ill with depressive disorder, or anxiety disorder, or bipolar disorder or borderline personality disorder. Asset-based community development[31] takes this further and may be promoted by primary care practitioners who can advocate for mental well-being as one of the outcomes alongside others, such as alleviation of poverty, generation of employment or reduction in violence. An example of these includes cash transfers to families with the aim of improving well-being and mental health of children.[38]

In conclusion, as HICs are now engaged in redesigning services and approaches to mental health care, an opportunity exists for LMICs to take a shortcut, revert to the principles of Alma Ata and develop primary care mental health systems which both support individuals to cope with distress and take on a whole population and community approach. Given the problems of the diagnostic system and the clear evidence that psychotropic medication has low effectiveness, clinicians can be reassured they do not need to escalate prescribing and can shift to a more radically open approach to information-sharing about the low likelihood of benefit, strong possibilities of side effects and withdrawal symptoms and uncertainties about long-term harm. It might also be important to be clear about the low effectiveness of psychotherapy and be aware that it could be prohibitively expensive if scaled up for all individuals with anxiety and depression. Therapy in groups[34] or that has wider systemic effects might be more important to develop, alongside supporting individuals to engage in social interventions addressing current adversity and supporting communities to reinforce natural instincts towards listening and kindness and to prevent violence.

REFERENCES

1. Summerfield D. How scientifically valid is the knowledge base of global mental health? BMJ. 2008;336:992–4. https://doi.org/10.1136/bmj.39513.441030.AD
2. Kessler RC, Ormel J, Petukhova M, et al. Development of lifetime comorbidity in the World Health Organization world mental health surveys. Arch Gen Psychiatry. 2011;68(1):90–100. https://doi.org/10.1001/archgenpsychiatry.2010.180
3. Pilgrim D, Bentall R. The medicalisation of misery: a critical realist analysis of the concept of depression. J Ment Health. 1999;8(3):261–74. https://doi.org/10.1080/0963823 9917427
4. Moncrieff J, Cooper RE, Stockmann T, Amendola S, Hengartner MP, Horowitz MA. The serotonin theory of depression: a systematic umbrella review of the evidence. Mol Psychiatry. 2022. https://doi.org/10.1038/s41380-022-01661-0
5. Shapiro MB. The social origins of depression: by G. W. Brown and T. Harris: its methodological philosophy. Behav Res Ther. 1979;17(6):597–603. https://doi.org/10.1016/0005-7967(79)90104-9
6. Anda RF, Felitti VJ, Bremner JD, et al. The enduring effects of abuse and related adverse experiences in childhood. A convergence of evidence from neurobiology and epidemiology. Eur Arch Psychiatry Clin Neurosci. 2006;256(3):174–86. https://doi.org/10.1007/s00406-005-0624-4
7. Danese A, Lewis SJ. Psychoneuroimmunology of early-life stress: the hidden wounds of childhood trauma? Neuropsychopharmacol. 2017;42(1):99–114. https://doi.org/10.1038/npp.2016.198
8. Craddock N, Owen MJ. The beginning of the end for the Kraepelinian dichotomy. Br J Psychiatry. 2018;186(5):364–6. https://doi.org/10.1192/bjp.186.5.364
9. Priest RG, Paykel ES, Hart D, Baldwin DS, Roberts A, Vize C. Progress in defeating depression. Psychiatric Bulletin. 1995;19(8):491–5. https://doi.org/10.1192/pb.19.8.491
10. O'Connor EA, Whitlock EP, Gaynes B, Beil TL. Screening for Depression in Adults and Older Adults in Primary Care: An Updated Systematic Review. Rockville (MD): Agency for Healthcare Research and Quality (US). Report No: 10-05143-EF-1. 2009. Available from: https://www.ncbi.nlm.nih.gov/books/NBK36403/
11. Karasz A, Dowrick C, Byng R, et al. What we talk about when we talk about depression: doctor-patient conversations and treatment decision outcomes. Br J Gen Pract. 2012;62(594):e55–e63. https://doi.org/10.3399/bjgp12X616373
12. Kvaale EP, Haslam N, Gottdiener WH. The 'side effects' of medicalization: a meta-analytic review of how biogenetic explanations affect stigma. Clin Psychol Rev. 2013;33(6):782–94. https://doi.org/10.1016/j.cpr.2013.06.002
13. The National Institute of Mental Health. Research Funded by NIMH. [cited 2023 April 21] Available from: NIMH » Research Funded by NIMH (https://www.nimh.nih.gov/research/research-funded-by-nimh/rdoc)
14. Saxe GN, Bickman L, Ma S, Aliferis C. Mental health progress requires causal diagnostic nosology and scalable causal discovery. Front Psychiatry. 2002;13:898789. https://doi.org/10.3389/fpsyt.2022.898789
15. Kotov R, Krueger RF, Watson D, et al. The Hierarchical Taxonomy of Psychopathology (HiTOP): a dimensional alternative to traditional nosologies. J Abnorm Psychol. 2017;126(4):454–77. https://doi.org/10.1037/abn0000258
16. Middleton H, Moncrieff J. Critical psychiatry: a brief overview. BJPysch Advances. 2019;25(1):47–54. https://doi.org/10.1192/bja.2018.38
17. Sartorius N. Fighting for Mental Health: A Personal View. Cambridge University Press; 2002.
18. World Health Organisation. Mental Health and Substance Use. [cited 2023 April 21] Available from: Mental Health and Substance Use (who.int)

19. Arroll B, Elley CR, Fishman T, et al. Antidepressants versus placebo for depression in primary care. Cochrane Database Syst Rev. 2009. https://doi.org/10.1002/14651858.cd007954

20. Herrman H, Patel V, Kieling C, et al. Time for united action on depression: a Lancet-World Psychiatric Association Commission. Lancet. 2022;399(10328):957–1022. https://doi.org/10.1016/s0140-6736(21)02141-3

21. Taylor S, Annand F, Burkinshaw, P, et al. Dependence and Withdrawal Associated with Some Prescribed Medicines: An Evidence Review. Public Health England, 2019. [cited 2023 April 21]. Available from: Taylor: Dependence and withdrawal associated with… - Google Scholar

22. Exasol. EXASOL analyzes: Research shows that over 64m prescriptions of antidepressants are dispensed per year in England. 2017. [cited 2023 April 21] Available from: Exasol Analyzes: Research shows that over 64m prescriptions of antidepressants are dispensed per year in England. | Exasol

23. Byng R. Should we, can we, halt the rise in prescribing for pain and distress? Br J Gen Pract. 2020;70(689):432–3. https://doi.org/10.3399/bjgp20X712217

24. Piggot HE. STAR*D: A tale and trail of bias. Ethical Human Psychology and Psychiatry (EHPP: An International Journal of Critical Inquiry). 2011;13(1), 6–28. https://doi.org/10.1891/1559-4343.13.1.6

25. Cuijpers P, Cristea IA, Karyotaki E, Reijnders M, Huibers MJ. How effective are cognitive behavior therapies for major depression and anxiety disorders? A meta-analytic update of the evidence. World Psychiatry. 2016;15(3):245–58. https://doi.org/10.1002%2Fwps.20346

26. Watkins ER, Taylor RS, Byng R, et al. Guided self-help concreteness training as an intervention for major depression in primary care: a Phase II randomized controlled trial. Psychol Med. 2012;42(7):1359–71. https://doi.org/10.1017/S0033291711002480

27. Gabbay MB, Ring A, Byng R, et al. Debt Counselling for Depression in Primary Care: an adaptive randomised controlled pilot trial (DeCoDer study). Health Technol Assess. 2017;21(35):1–164. https://doi.org/10.3310/hta21350

28. World Health Organisation. WHO called to return to the Declaration of Alma-Ata. [cited 2023 April 21] Available from: Declaration of Alma-Ata (who.int)

29. Huxley P. Mental illness in the community: the Goldberg-Huxley model of the pathway to psychiatric care. Nord J Psychiatry. 2009;50(37):47–53. https://doi.org/10.3109/08039489609099730

30. Tudor Hart J. The inverse care law. Lancet. 1971;297(7696):405–12. https://doi.org/10.1016/S0140-6736(71)92410-X

31. What is Asset Based Community Development (ACD). [cited 2023 April 21] Available from: What is Asset Based Community Development (ABCD) Handout) (depaul.edu)

32. The DESTRESS project. [cited 2023 April 21] Available from: DeSTRESS Project – Understanding and Dealing with Stress

33. Bolton P, Lee C, Haroz EE, et al. A transdiagnostic community-based mental health treatment for comorbid disorders: development and outcomes of a randomized controlled trial among Burmese refugees in Thailand. PLoS Med. 2014;11(11):e1001757. https://doi.org/10.1371/journal.pmed.1001757

34. Bolton P, Bass J, Neugebauer R, et al. Group interpersonal psychotherapy for depression in rural Uganda: a randomized controlled trial. JAMA. 2003;289(23):3117–24. https://doi.org/10.1001/jama.289.23.3117

35. Strong Minds. Our Results: Ending the Depression Epidemic in Africa. [cited 2023 April 21] Available from: OUR IMPACT - StrongMinds

36. Murray LK, Kane JC, Glass N, et al. Effectiveness of the Common Elements Treatment Approach (CETA) in reducing intimate partner violence and hazardous alcohol use in Zambia (VATU): a randomized controlled trial. PLoS Med. 2020;17(4):e1003056. https://doi.org/10.1371/journal.pmed.1003056

37. NHS England. The Community Mental Health Framework for Adults and Older Adults. (2019) [cited 2023 April 21]. Available from: https://www.england.nhs.uk/publication/the-community-mental-health-framework-for-adults-and-older-adults/

38. Zimmerman A, Garman E, Avendano-Pabon M, et al. The impact of cash transfers on mental health in children and young people in low-income and middle-income countries: a systematic review and meta-analysis. BMJ Glob Health. 2021;6(4):e004661. https://doi.org/10.1136/bmjgh-2020-004661

CHAPTER 3

Assessment for depression and anxiety in primary care

DOI: 10.1201/9781003391531-3

3.1 THE CASE FOR AND AGAINST SCREENING

Felicity Goodyear-Smith

There is an argument that screening for conditions such as depression and anxiety may confer benefits. Patients with these conditions are identified, ideally early in their disease trajectory, and offered appropriate treatment and care. However, there are also potential harms from mass screening of populations. No test is 100% sensitive or specific. There will be false negatives, meaning that some people with the conditions may be missed. There will also be false positives, whereby people who are not truly clinically depressed or anxious are wrongly diagnosed. Effective evidence-based management also needs to be available and cost-effective within the available health system.

CRITERIA FOR SCREENING

The World Health Organization (WHO) identifies the following criteria to justify screening:[1]

1. The condition sought should be an important health problem.
2. There should be an accepted treatment for patients with recognised disease.
3. Facilities for diagnosis and treatment should be available.
4. There should be a recognisable latent or early symptomatic stage.
5. There should be a suitable test or examination.
6. The test should be acceptable to the population.
7. The natural history of the condition, including development from latent to declared disease, should be adequately understood.
8. There should be an agreed policy on whom to treat as patients.
9. The cost of case-finding (including diagnosis and treatment of patients diagnosed) should be economically balanced in relation to possible expenditure on medical care as a whole.
10. Case-finding should be a continuing process and not a 'once and for all' project.

The *Journal of the American Medical Association* (JAMA) evidence-based medicine working group recommendations[2] outline similar factors to be considered:

Are the recommendations valid?

- Is there randomised controlled trial (RCT) evidence that earlier intervention works?
- Were the data identified, selected, and combined in an unbiased fashion?

What are the recommendations, and will they help you in caring for your patients?

- What are the benefits?
- What are the harms?
- How do benefits and harms compare in different people and with different screening strategies?
- What is the impact of people's values and preferences?
- What is the impact of uncertainty associated with the evidence?
- What is the cost-effectiveness?

Effectively, two criteria should be met: There must be an accurate test for the condition, and there must be scientific evidence that screening can prevent adverse outcomes. The test must be able to detect the target condition earlier than without screening and with sufficient accuracy to avoid producing large numbers of false-positive and false-negative results. Screening for, and treating persons with, early disease should improve the likelihood of favourable health outcomes (for example, disease-specific morbidity or mortality) compared with treating patients when they present with signs or symptoms of disease. Ultimately, an RCT needs to be performed to verify this claim.

Screening and case-finding

Screening tests do not diagnose an illness. Those testing positive need to undergo a 'gold-standard' diagnostic test. Screening tests should have a good sensitivity (identify most people with the condition) and adequate specificity (identify most people who do not have the condition). However, there is a risk that there will be false negatives, and hence underdiagnosis, but also false positives and hence overinvestigation, overdiagnosis, or misdiagnosis.

The terms screening and case-finding are sometimes used synonymously.[3] However, while both involve the early detection of a condition, there is a range from a broad-based programme through to opportunistic screening of an individual. Mass screening involves testing an asymptomatic population for the presence of a condition, which, if identified, can led to early intervention, reducing subsequent morbidity or mortality. This is usually conducted by inviting the target population to attend for testing. For a specific condition, testing will depend on a number of criteria, including the age and gender of the patient. Examples include breast and cervical cancer screening for eligible women. However, when an entire population is screened, for most conditions, it will be expected that the vast majority will be negative (do not have the disease). The smaller the likelihood of a screened person having a condition (i.e., a low pre-test probability), the greater the risk that they will have a false-positive result, meaning they will need to undergo unnecessary investigations.

If the screening is targeted to a specific population beyond demographics such as age or sex, this problem may be reduced. People might only be eligible for screening if they have certain risk factors which increase their likelihood of being a positive case (i.e., the pre-test probability is increased). These factors might be genetic variants, having another health condition or lifestyle factors – for example, screening smokers for lung cancer.

Case-finding may be considered to be offering a screening test opportunistically to an individual, although there is no clearcut definitions of 'screening' and 'case-finding'. Case-finding in a primary care consultation may involve seeking early detection of a condition when a patient attends for an unrelated concurrent disorder, who may or may not be symptomatic.

SHOULD WE SCREEN FOR DEPRESSION AND ANXIETY?

A number of systematic reviews and meta-analyses have been conducted on screening for depression, using the accepted criteria noted earlier. Three conducted by Gilbody and colleagues between 2001 and 2008, including one Cochrane review, did not favour screening.[3–5] On the other hand, two reviews by the US Preventive Services Task Force (USPTF) in 2002[6,7] and 2009[8,9] favoured screening. An analysis exploring these opposing recommendations found that a major factor was whether a review included or excluded a large study which provided data on the outcome of the effect of depression screening on treatment (i.e., whether the patient received treatment for depression).[10]

Assessment of these differing reviews demonstrates how decisions in the meta-analysis process can shape the conclusion. This study shows that even meta-analyses are never value-free.[11] While scientific enquiry extends empirical knowledge and directs evidence-based practice, research findings are neither complete nor immutable and will always rest on the questions we ask and the interpretations we make.[12] Application of generic findings needs to be contextualised. The decision to screen or not to screen depends on many context-specific factors, in particular the availability and accessibility of effective interventions.

In his chapter on alternative models of care, Richard Byng challenges the dominant view that depression and anxiety should be approached as diseases or disorders which need detecting and treating. From his perspective, common mental problems occur in every community as people struggle to meet the social and psychological issues in their life journeys. Given the heterogenous symptom clusters, for example, sleeping or eating too much or too little, being slow or agitated, he argues that often diagnostic labels are applied inappropriately. Further, the effect sizes for both pharmaceutical and psychological interventions are small, and he advocates an approach focused on supporting individuals to cope with distress. Under his paradigm, use of screening tools in primary care does not meet the criterion that 'there is RCT evidence that earlier intervention works'.

REFERENCES

1. Wilson JM, Jungler G. Principles and practice of screening for disease. Geneva: World Health Organization 1968:163.
2. Barratt A, Irwig L, Glasziou P, et al. Users' guides to the medical literature: XVII. How to use guidelines and recommendations about screening. Evidence-Based Medicine Working Group. JAMA. 1999;281(21):2029–34.
3. Gilbody S, Sheldon T, House A. Screening and case-finding instruments for depression: a meta-analysis. Can Med Assoc J. 2008;178(8):997–1003.
4. Gilbody S, House AO, Sheldon TA. Screening and case finding instruments for depression. Cochrane Database Syst Rev. 2019; 2005(4):CD002792.
5. Gilbody SM, House AO, Sheldon TA. Routinely administered questionnaires for depression and anxiety: systematic review. BMJ. 2001;322(7283):406–9.
6. Pignone MP, Gaynes BN, Rushton JL, et al. Screening for depression in adults: a summary of the evidence for the U.S. Preventive Services Task Force. Ann Intern Med. 2002;136(10):765–76.
7. Anonymous. Summaries for patients. Screening for depression: recommendations from the U.S. Preventive Services Task Force. [Original report in Ann Intern Med. 2002;136(10):765–76; PMID: 12020146]. [Original report in Ann Intern Med. 2002;136(10):760–4; PMID: 12020145]. Ann Intern Med. 2002;136(10):I56.
8. O'Connor EA, Whitlock EP, Beil TL, et al. Screening for depression in adult patients in primary care settings: a systematic evidence review. Ann Intern Med. 2009;151(11):793–803.
9. Anonymous. Summaries for patients. Screening for depression in adults: U.S. preventive services task force recommendations. Ann Intern Med. 2009;151(11):I56.
10. Wells KB, Sherbourne C, Schoenbaum M, et al. Impact of disseminating quality improvement programs for depression in managed primary care: a randomized controlled trial. [Erratum appears in JAMA 2000;283(24):3204]. JAMA. 2000; 283(2):212–20.
11. Goodyear-Smith FA, van Driel ML, Arroll B, et al. Analysis of decisions made in meta-analyses of depression screening and the risk of confirmation bias: a case study. BMC Med Res Methodol. 2012;12:76. doi: http://dx.doi.org/10.1186/1471-2288-12-76
12. Goodyear-Smith F. Practising alchemy: the transmutation of evidence into best health care Fam Pract. 2011;28(2):123–27. doi: 10.1093/fampra/cmq106

3.2 TOOLS USED FOR ASSESSING AND SCREENING FOR DEPRESSION AND ANXIETY IN PRIMARY CARE

Sherina Mohd Sidik and Felicity Goodyear-Smith

In the previous two chapters, we have discussed screening our clinical populations for depression and anxiety. It can be seen that, at least in primary care settings, where these conditions are likely to be less severe than in secondary-care psychiatric patient populations, there is a lack of consensus as to whether these conditions should be screened for and diagnosed.

However, there are in fact many mental health assessment and screening tools available and used in primary care. In this chapter we review the most commonly used tools for assessing depression and anxiety in primary care settings.

In 2018 a systemic literature review identified and evaluated publicly available, psychometrically tested tools that primary care physicians can use to screen adult patients for common mental disorders such as depression, anxiety and substance misuse.[1] The review identified 24 tools that screen for behavioural health disorders in adults in primary care settings. There were 13 short instruments with five or fewer items and 11 longer instruments. Sixteen of these 24 were unique tools, and 8 were subscales or portions of subscales originally developed as part of the longer instruments. Some were single-disorder tools (including four for substance use disorders), and some were multi-disorder, assessing for more than one mental health or substance use disorder. This chapter focuses on mental health disorders and does not discuss tools solely assessing substance misuse.

TOOLS FOR SCREENING DEPRESSION IN PRIMARY CARE
Patient Health Questionnaire (PHQ)

The Patient Health Questionnaire (PHQ) is the most tested and commonly used depression-screening tool in primary care settings. The PHQ-9 is a self-report tool, consisting of nine questions based on the nine *Diagnostic and Statistical Manual of Mental Disorders, Fifth Edition* (DSM-V) criteria for major depression, and is used to determine the presence or absence of depression (Figure 3.1).[2] PHQ-9 scores range from 0 to 27, as each of the nine items are scored from 0 (not at all) to 3 (nearly every day). PHQ-9 scores of 5, 10, 15, and 20 represent mild, moderate, moderately severe, and severe depression, respectively Although a screening tool, it is sometimes used for making diagnoses, for assessing severity of depressive disorders, and for monitoring treatment.

Over the *last 2 weeks*, how often have you been bothered by the following problems?	Not at all	Several days	More than half the days	Nearly every day
1. Little interest or pleasure in doing things	0	+1	+2	+3
2. Feeling down, depressed or hopeless	0	+1	+2	+3
3. Trouble falling asleep, staying asleep, or sleeping too much	0	+1	+2	+3
4. Feeling tired or having little energy	0	+1	+2	+3
5. Poor appetite or overeating	0	+1	+2	+3
6. Feeling bad about yourself – or that you're a failure or have let yourself or your family down	0	+1	+2	+3
7. Trouble concentrating on things, such as reading the newspaper or watching television	0	+1	+2	+3
8. Moving or speaking so slowly that other people could have noticed. Or, the opposite – being so fidgety or restless that you have been moving around a lot more than usual	0	+1	+2	+3
9. Thoughts that you would be better off dead or of hurting yourself in some way	0	+1	+2	+3

Interpretation:

- Total score of 5, 10, 15, and 20 represent cut-off points for mild, moderate, moderately severe, and severe depression, respectively.
- Note: Question 9 is a single screening question on suicide risk. A patient who answers yes to question 9 needs further assessment for suicide risk by an individual who is competent to assess this risk.

Provisional Diagnosis and Proposed Treatment Actions

PHQ-9 Score	Depression Severity	Proposed Treatment Actions
0–4	None-minimal	None
5–9	Mild	Watchful waiting; repeat PHQ-9 at follow-up
10–14	Moderate	Treatment plan, considering counselling, follow-up and/or pharmacotherapy
15–19	Moderately severe	Active treatment with pharmacotherapy and/or psychotherapy
20–27	Severe	Immediate initiation of pharmacotherapy and, if severe impairment or poor response to therapy, expedited referral to a mental health specialist for psychotherapy and/or collaborative management

FIGURE 3.1 Patient Health Questionnaire (PHQ-9).

Its validity as a brief depression severity measure was first published in 2001, where at a score of 10 and above, the PHQ-9 had a high sensitivity of 88% and specificity of 88% for major depression.[3] The PHQ-9 has been translated into many different languages and has widespread use globally. Validation and calibration studies have been conducted in many countries including Argentina,[4] Bangladesh,[5] Columbia,[6] Tunisia,[7] Malaysia,[8] and New Zealand.[9]

There are a number of PHQ sub-scales that can be administered and scored separately. The PHQ-8 consists of eight of the nine criteria based on the DSM-IV diagnosis of depressive disorders, where the ninth question of the PHQ-9, which assesses suicidal or self-injurious thoughts, has been omitted. It has been found to be comparable to the PHQ-9 in terms of diagnosing depressive disorders, with a cut-point $\geq$10 used for defining current depression.[10]

The ultra-brief PHQ-2 comprises the first two questions and is often used for a rapid initial assessment. A PHQ-2 threshold score of 3 has been found to have a sensitivity of 74% and specificity of 60% for a diagnosis of major depressive illness.[11] It is indicated as a useful and efficient screener and measure of treatment progress and outcomes in routine primary care.[12] Adding a 'help' question to the PHQ-2, asking whether the person would like help either immediately or at a later time, found a general practitioner diagnosis with a 79% sensitivity and a 94% specificity.[13]

A large validation study of the PHQ-2 and PHQ-9 in primary care found that the sensitivity and specificity of the PHQ-2 for diagnosing major depression were 86% and 78%, respectively, with a score of 2 or higher and 61% and 92% with a score 3 or higher. For the PHQ-9, they were 74% and 91%, respectively, with a score of 10 or higher.[14]

Hamilton Depression Rating Scale (HAM-D)

An early screening tool for depression is the Hamilton Depression Rating Scale (HAM-D), developed in 1960. The original version contains 17 items (HAM-D$_{17}$ or HDRS17) pertaining to symptoms of depression experienced over the past week (Figure 3.2).[15] The HDRS was originally developed for hospital inpatients to assess severity and change in depressive symptoms in adults. A score of 0–7 is generally accepted to be within the normal range (or in clinical remission), while a score of 20 or higher indicates at least moderate severity.

There are a number of different versions of varying lengths: HAM-D$_6$, HAM-D$_7$, HAM-D$_8$, HAM-D$_{21}$, HAM-D$_{24}$, and HAM-D$_{29}$, as well as an Interactive Voice Response version (IVR), a Seasonal Affective Disorder version, and a Structured Interview Version (HDS-SIV).[16] The HAM-D is

PLEASE COMPLETE THE SCALE BASED ON A STRUCTURED INTERVIEW

Instructions: For each item select the one "cue" which best characterizes the patient. Be sure to record the answers in the appropriate spaces (positions 0–4).

1. **DEPRESSED MOOD** (sadness, hopeless, helpless, worthless)
   0 |__| Absent.
   1 |__| These feeling states indicated only on questioning.
   2 |__| These feeling states spontaneously reported verbally.
   3 |__| Communicates feeling states non-verbally, i.e., through facial expression, posture, voice and tendency to weep.
   4 |__| Patient reports virtually only these feeling states in his/her spontaneous verbal and non-verbal communication.

2. **FEELINGS OF GUILT**
   0 |__| Absent.
   1 |__| Self-reproach, feels he/she has let people down.
   2 |__| Ideas of guilt or rumination over past errors or sinful deeds.
   3 |__| Present illness is a punishment. Delusions of guilt.
   4 |__| Hears accusatory or denunciatory voices and/or experiences threatening visual hallucinations.

3. **SUICIDE**
   0 |__| Absent.
   1 |__| Feels life is not worth living.
   2 |__| Wishes he/she were dead or any thoughts of possible death to self.
   3 |__| Ideas or gestures of suicide.
   4 |__| Attempts at suicide (any serious attempt rate 4).

4. **INSOMNIA: EARLY IN THE NIGHT**
   0 |__| No difficulty falling asleep.
   1 |__| Complains of occasional difficulty falling asleep, i.e., more than half an hour.
   2 |__| Complains of nightly difficulty falling asleep.

5. **INSOMNIA: MIDDLE OF THE NIGHT**
   0 |__| No difficulty.
   1 |__| Patient complains of being restless and disturbed during the night.
   2 |__| Waking during the night – any getting out of bed rates 2 (except for purposes of voiding).

6. **INSOMNIA: EARLY HOURS OF THE MORNING**
   0 |__| No difficulty.
   1 |__| Waking in early hours of the morning but goes back to sleep.
   2 |__| Unable to fall asleep again if he/she gets out of bed.

7. **WORK AND ACTIVITIES**
   0 |__| No difficulty.
   1 |__| Thoughts and feelings of incapacity, fatigue or weakness related to activities, work or hobbies.
   2 |__| Loss of interest in activity, hobbies, or work – either directly reported by the patient or indirect in listlessness, indecision, and vacillation (feels he/she has to push self to work or activities).
   3 |__| Decrease in actual time spent in activities or decrease in productivity. Rate 3 if the patient does not spend at least three hours a day in activities (job or hobbies) excluding routine chores.
   4 |__| Stopped working because of present illness. Rate 4 if patient engages in no activities except routine chores, or if patient fails to perform routine chores unassisted.

8. **RETARDATION** (slowness of thought and speech, impaired ability to concentrate, decreased motor activity)
   0 |__| Normal speech and thought.
   1 |__| Slight retardation during the interview.
   2 |__| Obvious retardation during the interview.
   3 |__| Interview difficult.
   4 |__| Complete stupor.

9. **AGITATION**
   0 |__| None.
   1 |__| Fidgetiness.
   2 |__| Playing with hands, hair, etc.
   3 |__| Moving about, can't sit still.
   4 |__| Hand wringing, nail biting, hair-pulling, biting of lips.

FIGURE 3.2 Hamilton Depression Rating Scale (HAM-D$_{17}$ or HDRS17).

(*Continued*)

10. **ANXIETY PSYCHIC**
    0 |__| No difficulty.
    1 |__| Subjective tension and irritability.
    2 |__| Worrying about minor matters.
    3 |__| Apprehensive attitude apparent in face or speech.
    4 |__| Fears expressed without questioning.

11. **ANXIETY SOMATIC (physiological concomitants of anxiety) such as:**
    gastrointestinal – dry mouth, wind, indigestion, diarrhoea, cramps, belching
    cardiovascular – palpitations, headaches
    respiratory – hyperventilation, sighing
    urinary frequency
    sweating
    0 |__| Absent.
    1 |__| Mild.
    2 |__| Moderate.
    3 |__| Severe.
    4 |__| Incapacitating.

12. **SOMATIC SYMPTOMS GASTROINTESTINAL**
    0 |__| None.
    1 |__| Loss of appetite but eating without staff encouragement. Heavy feelings in abdomen.
    2 |__| Difficulty eating without staff urging. Requests or requires laxatives or medication for bowels or medication for gastrointestinal symptoms.

13. **GENERAL SOMATIC SYMPTOMS**
    0 |__| None.
    1 |__| Heaviness in limbs, back, or head. Backaches, headaches, muscle aches. Loss of energy and fatigability.
    2 |__| Any clear-cut symptom rates 2.

14. **GENITAL SYMPTOMS** (symptoms such as loss of libido, menstrual disturbances)
    0 |__| Absent.
    1 |__| Mild.
    2 |__| Severe.

15. **HYPOCHONDRIASIS**
    0 |__| Not present.
    1 |__| Self-absorption (bodily).
    2 |__| Preoccupation with health.
    3 |__| Frequent complaints, requests for help, etc.
    4 |__| Hypochondriacal delusions.

16. **LOSS OF WEIGHT (RATE EITHER a OR b)**

a) According to the patients:	**b) According to weekly measurements:**
0 |__| No weight loss.	0 |__| Less than 1 lb weight loss in week.
1 |__| Probable weight loss associated with present illness.	1 |__| Greater than 1 lb weight loss in week.
2 |__| Definite (according to patient) weight loss.	2 |__| Greater than 2 lb weight loss in week.
3 |__| Not assessed.	3 |__| Not assessed.

17. **INSIGHT**
    0 |__| Acknowledges being depressed and ill.
    1 |__| Acknowledges illness but attributes cause to bad food, climate, overwork, virus, need for rest, etc.
    2 |__| Denies being ill at all.

Total score: |__|__|

This scale is in the public domain.

FIGURE 3.2 (*Continued*)

often used as a research tool but has limited use in primary care and was not included in Mulvaney-Day et al.'s systematic review.[1]

Beck Depression Inventory (BDI-II)

The Beck Depression Inventory (BDI) is a self-report tool developed in 1961 to measure the severity of depression.[17] The BDI was revised to include additional items and reflect changes in the DSM. The revised vBDI, known as the BDI-II, is the most widely used version and includes 21 items, each of which corresponds to a symptom of depression. For the BDI-II, a score of 10–18 indicates mild depression and ≥30 indicates severe depression.[18] The BDI has good reliability and validity. The test-retest reliability of the BDI-II ranged from 0.73 to 0.92, which means that the scores are consistent over time. The internal consistency of the BDI-II was 0.9, which means that the items on the questionnaire relate to each other and measure the same construct.[1]

Although the BDI-II was previously endorsed by the National Institute for Health and Clinical Excellence (NICE) for use in primary care to measure baseline depression severity and treatment responsiveness,[18] it is predominantly a research tool. Furthermore the official BDI is copyrighted and must be purchased for use; hence, the freely available PHQ-9 is a preferable primary care choice.

Edinburgh Postnatal Depression Scale (EPDS)

The Edinburgh Postnatal Depression Scale (EPDS) is a specific tool used only for women during pregnancy and for the first 12 months after delivery to identify those at risk for perinatal depression.[6,7] The 10-question tool assesses depressive symptoms for the past seven days, with those scoring >13 likely to be suffering from a depressive illness of varying severity (Figure 3.3).[19] An early study found that using a cut-off value of ≥5 gave a sensitivity of 71% and specificity of 65%,[20] but in a more recent and larger study, the optimal cut-off score during the second trimester was seen to be 4/5, with a sensitivity of 86% and specificity of 77%.[21] Using the ≥5 cut-off value may be adequate for initial screening, followed by further assessments and possibly antenatal intervention when positive.[22]

TOOLS FOR SCREENING ANXIETY IN PRIMARY CARE
Generalized Anxiety Disorder Questionnaire (GAD-7)

The seven-item Generalized Anxiety Disorder scale (GAD-7) was developed for use in primary care (Figure 3.4).[23,24] It is a self-reported tool with

Name:_____   Address: _____

Your Date of Birth: _____   _____

Baby's Date of Birth: _____   Phone: _____

As you are pregnant or have recently had a baby, we would like to know how you are feeling. Please check the answer that comes closest to how you have felt IN THE PAST 7 DAYS, not just how you feel today. Here is an example, already completed.

☐ I have felt happy: This would mean: "I have felt happy most
☐ Yes, all the time   of the time" during the past week.
☒ Yes, most of the time   Please complete the other questions in the
☐ No, not very often   same way.
☐ No, not at all

In the past 7 days:

1. I have been able to laugh and see the funny side of things
   ☐ As much as I always could
   ☐ Not quite so much now to cope at all
   ☐ Definitely not so much now
   ☐ Not at all
2. I have looked forward with enjoyment to things
   ☐ As much as I ever did
   ☐ Rather less than I used to
   ☐ Definitely less than I used to
   ☐ Hardly at all
3. I have blamed myself unnecessarily when things went wrong
   ☐ Yes, most of the time
   ☐ Yes, some of the time
   ☐ Not very often
   ☐ No, never
4. I have been anxious or worried for no good reason
   ☐ No, not at all
   ☐ Hardly ever
   ☐ Yes, sometimes
   ☐ Yes, very often
5. I have felt scared or panicky for no very good reason
   ☐ Yes, quite a lot
   ☐ Yes, sometimes
   ☐ No, not much
   ☐ No, not at all

6. Things have been getting on top of me
   ☐ Yes, most of the time I haven't been able to cope at all
   ☐ Yes, sometimes I haven't been coping as well as usual
   ☐ No, most of the time I have coped quite well
   ☐ No, I have been coping as well as ever
7. I have been so unhappy that I have had difficulty sleeping
   ☐ Yes, most of the time
   ☐ Yes, sometimes
   ☐ Not very often
   ☐ No, not at all
8. I have felt sad or miserable
   ☐ Yes, most of the time
   ☐ Yes, quite often
   ☐ Not very often
   ☐ No, not at all
9. I have been so unhappy that I have been crying
   ☐ Yes, most of the time
   ☐ Yes, quite often
   ☐ Only occasionally
   ☐ No, never
10. The thought of harming myself has occurred to me
    ☐ Yes, quite often
    ☐ Sometimes
    ☐ Hardly ever
    ☐ Never

FIGURE 3.3 Edinburgh Postnatal Depression Scale (EPDS). (*Continued*)

SCORING
QUESTIONS 1, 2, AND 4 (without an *)
Are scored 0, 1, 2, or 3 with the top box scored as 0 and the bottom box scored as 3.

QUESTIONS 3, 5–10 (marked with an *)
Are reverse-scored, with the top box scored as a 3 and the bottom box scored as 0.

Maximum score: 30
Possible depression: 10 or greater
Always look at item 10 (suicidal thoughts)

Users may reproduce the scale without further permission, providing they respect copyright by quoting the names of the authors, the title, and the source of the paper in all reproduced copies.

Instructions for using the Edinburgh Postnatal Depression Scale:

1. The mother is asked to check the response that comes closest to how she has been feeling in the previous 7 days.
2. All the items must be completed.
3. Care should be taken to avoid the possibility of the mother discussing her answers with others. (Answers come from the mother or pregnant woman.)
4. The mother should complete the scale herself, unless she has limited English or has difficulty with reading.

FIGURE 3.3 *(Continued)*

demonstrated good reliability with a sensitivity for diagnosing anxiety (cut-off point ≥8) of 92% and specificity of 76%. It can therefore be used to determine the presence or absence of anxiety at a recommended cut-off point of 8 and above, although scores of 5, 10, and 15 are taken as the cut-off points for mild, moderate, and severe anxiety, respectively.[24] Apart from detecting GAD, the GAD-7 can also detect panic disorder, social anxiety disorder, and post-traumatic stress disorder (PTSD), and is most appropriate for use in primary care settings.[23] The seven items refer to symptoms experienced during the two weeks prior to answering the questionnaire, and each item has four answers ("not at all", "several days", "more than half the days", and "nearly every day"), scored from 0 (not at all) to 3 (nearly every day). Scores of GAD-7 range from 0 to 21.

The GAD-7 has widespread use and has been validated in a number of different countries and settings, including Malaysia,[25] Cyprus,[26] and Korea.[27]

The GAD-2 is an ultra-quick version, consisting of the first two questions of the GAD-7. It has been validated in a number of studies and has been proposed as a first step for screening for GAD[28] and measuring treatment progress and outcomes in routine clinical care.[12]

Over the *last 2 weeks*, how often have you been bothered by the following problems?	Not at all	Several days	More than half the days	Nearly every day
1. Feeling nervous, anxious, or on edge	0	+1	+2	+3
2. Not being able to stop or control worrying	0	+1	+2	+3
3. Worrying too much about different things	0	+1	+2	+3
4. Trouble relaxing	0	+1	+2	+3
5. Being so restless that i is hard to sit still	0	+1	+2	+3
6. Becoming easily annoyed or irritable	0	+1	+2	+3
7. Feeling afraid, as if something awful might happen	0	+1	+2	+3

Column totals: _____ + _____ + _____ + _____

Total score: _____

If you checked any problems, how difficult have they made it for you to do your work, take care of things at home, or get along with other people?

Not difficult at all	Somewhat difficult	Very difficult	Extremely difficult
☐	☐	☐	☐

Scoring GAD-7 Anxiety Severity
This is calculated by assigning scores of 0, 1, 2, and 3 to the response categories, respectively, of "not at all," "several days," "more than half the days," and "nearly every day."

GAD-7 total score for the seven items ranges from 0 to 21.
0–4: minimal anxiety
5–9: mild anxiety
10–14: moderate anxiety
15–21: severe anxiety

FIGURE 3.4 Generalized Anxiety Disorder Scale (GAD-7).

TOOLS MEASURING STRESS AND DISTRESS
Kessler Psychological Distress Scale 10 (K10)

The Kessler Psychological Distress Scale (K10) is a simple measure of non-specific psychological distress (Figure 3.5).[29] The K10 scale involves 10 questions asking respondents how frequently they experienced symptoms of psychological distress (e.g., "feeling so sad that nothing can cheer you up")

Please tick the answer that is correct for you:	All of the time (score 5)	Most of the time (score 4)	Some of the time (score 3)	A little of the time (score 2)	None of the time (score 1)
1. In the past 4 weeks, about how often did you feel tired out for no good reason?					
2. In the past 4 weeks, about how often did you feel nervous?					
3. In the past 4 weeks, about how often did you feel so nervous that nothing could calm you down?					
4. In the past 4 weeks, about how often did you feel hopeless?					
5. In the past 4 weeks, about how often did you feel restless or fidgety?					
6. In the past 4 weeks, about how often did you feel so restless you could not sit still?					
7. In the past 4 weeks, about how often did you feel depressed?					
8. In the past 4 weeks, about how often did you feel that everything was an effort?					
9. In the past 4 weeks, about how often did you feel so sad that nothing could cheer you up?					
10. In the past 4 weeks, about how often did you feel worthless?					

In the context of injury management, the measure can be provided to the patient where recovery is not proceeding as anticipated (for instance, between weeks four and six) and may highlight the need for more regular review or referral to a specialist health provider such as a psychologist. Questions 3 and 6 do not need to be asked if the response to the preceding question was 'none of the time'. In such cases, questions 3 and 6 should receive an automatic score of 1.

FIGURE 3.5 Kessler Psychological Distress Scale (K10). (*Continued*)

Scoring instructions

Each item is scored from 1 'none of the time' to 5 'all of the time'. Scores of the 10 items are then summed, yielding a minimum score of 10 and a maximum score of 50. Low scores indicate low levels of psychological distress, and high scores indicate high levels of psychological distress.

Interpretation of scores

The 2001 Victorian Population Health Survey adopted a set of cut-off scores that may be used as a guide for screening for psychological distress. These are outlined next:

K10 Score: Likelihood of having a mental disorder (psychological distress)

10–19 Likely to be well
20–24 Likely to have a mild disorder
25–29 Likely to have a moderate disorder
30–50 Likely to have a severe disorder

FIGURE 3.5 (*Continued*)

during the past 30 days. Responses are recorded using a five-category scale (all of the time, most of the time, some of the time, a little of the time, and none of the time). This measure can be used as a brief screening tool to identify levels of distress. It can be self-completed, or alternatively, the questions can be read to the patient by the practitioner. Data from the Australia National Survey of Mental Health and Well-being (1997) found that there was a strong association between a high score of K10 and a current Composite International Diagnostic Interview (CIDI) diagnosis of anxiety or affective disorders.[30] The K6 has a subset of six of the questions.

Although it has been used in many countries, use of K6/K10 as a screening tool in culturally diverse populations is relatively untested.[31] When cut-off scores have not been validated in a local population, it is difficult to interpret the significance of a patient's score in a clinical setting. A high score should be taken seriously, as it may indicate mental health issues, but scores should not be taken at face value in populations where there has been no validation conducted and should be followed up with a clinical interview.

Perceived Stress Scale (PSS)

The original Perceived Stress Scale (PSS) was developed in 1983 as a 14-item scale (PSS-14) with 7 positive items and 7 negative items rated on a 5-point Likert scale (Figure 3.6).[32] It was shortened to the 10-item (PSS-10) and again to the 4-item (PSS-4). Psychometrically, the PSS-10 appears to be the best version to measure perceived stress, both in practice and in research.[33]

The Perceived Stress Scale (PSS) is a classic stress assessment instrument. The tool, while originally developed in 1983, remains a popular choice for helping us understand how different situations affect our feelings and our perceived stress. The questions in this scale ask about your feelings and thoughts during the last month. In each case, you will be asked to indicate how often you felt or thought a certain way. Although some of the questions are similar, there are differences between them, and you should treat each one as a separate question. The best approach is to answer fairly quickly. That is, don't try to count up the number of times you felt a particular way; rather, indicate the alternative that seems like a reasonable estimate.

For each question choose from the following alternatives:

In the last month:	Never 0	Almost never 1	Some-times 2	Fairly often 3	Very often 4
1. How often have you been upset because of something that happened unexpectedly?					
2. How often have you felt that you were unable to control the important things in your life?					
3. How often have you felt nervous and stressed?					
4. How often have you felt confident about your ability to handle your personal problems?					
5. How often have you felt that things were going your way?					
6. How often have you found that you could not cope with all the things that you had to do?					
7. How often have you been able to control irritations in your life?					
8. How often have you felt that you were on top of things?					
9. How often have you been angered because of things that happened that were outside of your control?					
10. How often have you felt difficulties were piling up so high that you could not overcome them?					

FIGURE 3.6 Perceived Stress Scale (PSS-10). (*Continued*)

Scoring

You can determine your PSS score by following these directions:

- First, reverse your scores for questions 4, 5, 7, and 8. On these four questions, change the scores like this: 0 = 4,   1 = 3,   2 = 2,   3 = 1,   4 = 0.
- Now add up your scores for each item to get a total. My total score is _____.
- Individual scores on the PSS can range from 0 to 40, with higher scores indicating higher perceived stress.

  ▶ Scores ranging from 0 to 13 would be considered low stress.
  ▶ Scores ranging from 14 to 26 would be considered moderate stress.
  ▶ Scores ranging from 27 to 40 would be considered high perceived stress.

The Perceived Stress Scale is interesting and important because your perception of what is happening in your life is most important. Consider the idea that two individuals could have the exact same events and experiences in their lives for the past month. Depending on their perception, the total score could put one of those individuals in the low stress category and the other person in the high stress category.

FIGURE 3.6 (*Continued*)

TOOLS COMBINING DEPRESSION AND ANXIETY SCREENING
Depression Anxiety and Stress Scale (DASS-21)

The DASS-21 is a short version (21 items) of a 42-item self-report tool designed to measure three related negative emotional states: depression (7 items), anxiety (7 items), and stress (7 items) (Figure 3.7).[34] Symptoms are scored on a 4-point Likert scale ranging from 0 ("Did not apply to me at all") to 3 ("Applied to me very much or most of the time"). DASS-21 has been found to have good convergent and discriminant validity when compared with other validated measures of depression and anxiety, such as the Hospital Anxiety and Depression Scale and the Personal Disturbance Scale.[35] The DASS-21 questionnaire is in the public domain and may be downloaded for use, with a scoring template and interpretation also available.

Patient Health Questionnaire 4 (PHQ-4)

The first two items from the PHQ-4, screening for depression, and the first two items from the GAD-7, screening for anxiety, have been combined into the PHQ-4.[36] This ultra-brief tool has been recommended as an efficient tool in settings with a strict limit in terms of time resources.

Please read each statement and circle a number 0, 1, 2, or 3 which indicates how much the statement applied to you over the past week. There are no right or wrong answers. Do not spend too much time on any statement.

The rating scale is as follows:
0. Did not apply to me at all
1. Applied to me to some degree, or some of the time
2. Applied to me to a considerable degree, or a good part of the time
3. Applied to me very much, or most of the time

1	I found it hard to wind down	0	1	2	3
2	I was aware of dryness of my mouth	0	1	2	3
3	I couldn't seem to experience any positive feeling at all	0	1	2	3
4	I experienced breathing difficulty (e.g., excessively rapid breathing, breathlessness in the absence of physical exertion)	0	1	2	3
5	I found it difficult to work up the initiative to do things	0	1	2	3
6	I tended to overreact to situations	0	1	2	3
7	I experienced trembling (e.g., in the hands)	0	1	2	3
8	I felt that I was using a lot of nervous energy	0	1	2	3
9	I was worried about situations in which I might panic and make a fool of myself	0	1	2	3
10	I felt that I had nothing to look forward to	0	1	2	3
11	I found myself getting agitated	0	1	2	3
12	I found it difficult to relax	0	1	2	3
13	I felt downhearted and blue	0	1	2	3
14	I was intolerant of anything that kept me from getting on with what I was doing	0	1	2	3
15	I felt I was close to panic	0	1	2	3
16	I was unable to become enthusiastic about anything	0	1	2	3
17	I felt I wasn't worth much as a person	0	1	2	3
18	I felt that I was rather touchy	0	1	2	3
19	I was aware of the action of my heart in the absence of physical exertion (e.g., sense of heart rate increase, heart missing a beat)	0	1	2	3
20	I felt scared without any good reason	0	1	2	3
21	I felt that life was meaningless	0	1	2	3

Totals

Interpreting DASS scores

	Depression	Anxiety	Stress
Normal	0–9	0–7	0–14
Mild	10–13	8–9	15–18
Moderate	14–20	10–14	19–25
Severe	21–27	15–19	26–33
Extremely severe	28+	20+	34+

FIGURE 3.7 Depression Anxiety Stress Scale (DASS 21).

The Mulvaney-Day et al. review found three ultra-short mental disorder tools screening for depression and anxiety: The Mental Health Inventory-5 (MHI-5),[37] the World Health Organization–Five Well-Being Index (WHO-5),[38] and the Brief Case-Find for Depression.[39] In general, these measures do not have strong sensitivity and specificity and are considered inferior to the PHQ-4.

CONCLUSION

It can be seen that there is a range of possible tools for primary care practitioners to use to detect depression, anxiety, or less specific 'distress' in their patient populations. In the following chapters, experts from a range of nations across the globe discuss the prevalence of these conditions in their respective countries, whether their populations are screened, and, if so, the tools they use and the types of interventions they offer positive cases. The authors of the country case studies were also asked whether they considered depression and anxiety to be useful diagnoses to make.

REFERENCES

1. Mulvaney-Day N, Marshall T, Downey Piscopo K, et al. Screening for behavioral health conditions in primary care settings: a systematic review of the literature. J Gen Intern Med. 2018;33(3):335–46. doi: 10.1007/s11606-017-4181-0 [published Online First: 2017/09/28]
2. Spitzer RL, Williams JB, Kroenke K, et al. Validity and utility of the PRIME-MD patient health questionnaire in assessment of 3000 obstetric-gynecologic patients: the PRIME-MD Patient Health Questionnaire Obstetrics-Gynecology Study. Am J Obstet Gynecol. 2000;183(3):759–69.
3. Kroenke K, Spitzer RL, Williams JB. The PHQ-9: validity of a brief depression severity measure. J Gen Intern Med. 2001;16(9):606–13.
4. Urtasun M, Daray FM, Teti GL, et al. Validation and calibration of the patient health questionnaire (PHQ-9) in Argentina. BMC Psychiatry. 2019;19(1):291. doi: 10.1186/s12888-019-2262-9
5. Naher R, Rabby MRA, Sharif F. Validation of patient health questionnaire-9 for assessing depression of adults in Bangladesh. Dhaka Univ J Biol Sci. 2021;30(2):275–81. doi: 10.3329/dujbs.v30i2.54652
6. Cassiani-Miranda CA, Cuadros-Cruz AK, Torres-Pinzón H, et al. Validity of the Patient Health Questionnaire-9 (PHQ-9) for depression screening in adult primary care users in Bucaramanga, Colombia. Rev Colomb Psiquiatr (Eng Ed). 2021;50(1):11–21. doi: 10.1016/j.rcpeng.2019.09.002
7. Belhadj H, Jomli R, Ouali U, et al. Validation of the Tunisian version of the patient health questionnaire (PHQ-9). Eur Psychiatry. 2017;41(S1):S523–S523. doi: 10.1016/j.eurpsy.2017.01.695 [published Online First: 2020/03/23]
8. Sherina MS, Arroll B, Goodyear-Smith F. Criterion validity of the PHQ-9 (Malay version) in a primary care clinic in Malaysia. Med J Malaysia. 2012;67(3):309–15. [published Online First: 2012/10/23]
9. Arroll B, Goodyear-Smith F, Crengle S, et al. Validation of PHQ-2 and PHQ-9 to screen for major depression in the primary care population. Ann Fam Med. 2010;8:348–53. doi: 10.1370/afm.1139

10. Kroenke K, Strine TW, Spitzer RL, et al. The PHQ-8 as a measure of current depression in the general population. J Affect Disord. 2009;114(1–3):163–73. doi: 10.1016/j.jad.2008.06.026 [published Online First: 2008/08/30]

11. Gelaye B, Wilson I, Berhane HY, et al. Diagnostic validity of the Patient Health Questionnaire-2 (PHQ-2) among Ethiopian adults. Compr Psychiatry. 2016;70:216–21. doi: 10.1016/j.comppsych.2016.07.011 [published Online First: 2016/08/28]

12. Staples LG, Dear BF, Gandy M, et al. Psychometric properties and clinical utility of brief measures of depression, anxiety, and general distress: the PHQ-2, GAD-2, and K-6. Gen Hosp Psychiatry. 2019;56:13–18. doi: 10.1016/j.genhosppsych.2018.11.003 [published Online First: 2018/12/07]

13. Arroll B, Goodyear-Smith F, Kerse N, et al. Effect of the addition of a "help" question to two screening questions on specificity for diagnosis of depression in general practice: diagnostic validity study. BMJ. 2005;331(7521):884.

14. Arroll B, Goodyear-Smith F, Crengle S, et al. Validation of PHQ-2 and PHQ-9 to screen for major depression in the primary care population. Ann Fam Med. 2010;8(4):348–53.

15. Hamilton M. A rating scale for depression. J Neurol Neurosurg Psychiatry. 1960;23(1): 56–62. doi: 10.1136/jnnp.23.1.56 [published online first: 1960/02/01]

16. Carrozzino D, Patierno C, Fava GA, et al. The Hamilton rating scales for depression: a critical review of clinimetric properties of different versions. Psychother Psychosom. 2020;89(3):133–50. doi: 10.1159/000506879 [published online first: 2020/04/15]

17. Beck AT. A systematic investigation of depression. Compr Psychiatry. 1961;2:163–70.

18. Smarr KL, Keefer AL. Measures of depression and depressive symptoms: beck Depression Inventory-II (BDI-II), Center for Epidemiologic Studies Depression Scale (CES-D), Geriatric Depression Scale (GDS), Hospital Anxiety and Depression Scale (HADS), and Patient Health Questionnaire-9 (PHQ-9). Arthritis Care Res. 2011;63(Suppl 11):S454–66. doi: 10.1002/acr.20556 [published online first: 2012/05/25]

19. Cox JL, Holden JM, Sagovsky R. Detection of postnatal depression. Development of the 10-item Edinburgh Postnatal Depression Scale. Br J Psychiatry. 1987;150:782–6. doi: 10.1192/bjp.150.6.782 [published online first: 1987/06/01]

20. Wisner KL, Parry BL, Piontek CM. Clinical practice. Postpartum depression. N Eng J Med. 2002;347(3):194–9. doi: 10.1056/NEJMcp011542 [published online first: 2002/07/19]

21. Tanuma-Takahashi A, Tanemoto T, Nagata C, et al. Antenatal screening timeline and cutoff scores of the Edinburgh Postnatal Depression Scale for predicting postpartum depressive symptoms in healthy women: a prospective cohort study. BMC Pregnancy Childbirth. 2022;22(1):527. doi: 10.1186/s12884-022-04740-w

22. Meijer JL, Beijers C, van Pampus MG, et al. Predictive accuracy of Edinburgh Postnatal Depression Scale assessment during pregnancy for the risk of developing postpartum depressive symptoms: a prospective cohort study. BJOG. 2014;121(13):1604–10. doi: https://doi.org/10.1111/1471-0528.12759

23. Kroenke K, Spitzer RL, Williams JBW, et al. Anxiety disorders in primary care: prevalence, impairment, comorbidity, and detection. Ann Intern Med. 2007;146(5):317–25.

24. Spitzer RL, Kroenke K, Williams JBW, et al. A brief measure for assessing generalized anxiety disorder: the GAD-7. Arch Intern Med. 2006;166(10):1092–7.

25. Sidik SM, Arroll B, Goodyear-Smith F. Validation of the GAD-7 (Malay version) among women attending a primary care clinic in Malaysia. J Prim Health Care. 2012;4(1):5–11, A1.

26. Vogazianos P, Motrico E, Domínguez-Salas S, et al. Validation of the generalized anxiety disorder screener (GAD-7) in Cypriot pregnant and postpartum women. BMC Pregnancy Childbirth. 2022;22(1):841. doi: 10.1186/s12884-022-05127-7

27. Lee B, Kim YE. The psychometric properties of the Generalized Anxiety Disorder scale (GAD-7) among Korean university students. Psychiatry Clin Psychopharmacol. 2019;29(4):864–71. doi: 10.1080/24750573.2019.1691320

28. Sapra A, Bhandari P, Sharma S, et al. Using Generalized Anxiety Disorder-2 (GAD-2) and GAD-7 in a primary care setting. Cureus. 2020;12(5):e8224. doi: 10.7759/cureus.8224 [published online first: 2020/06/26]

29. Kessler RC, Barker PR, Colpe LJ, et al. Screening for serious mental illness in the general population. Arch Gen Psychiatry. 2003;60(2):184–9. doi: 10.1001/archpsyc.60.2.184 [published online first: 2003/02/13]

30. Andrews G, Slade T. Interpreting scores on the Kessler Psychological Distress Scale (K10). Aus N Z J Public Health. 2001;25(6):494–97. doi: https://doi.org/10.1111/j.1467-842X.2001.tb00310.x

31. Stolk Y, Kaplan I, Szwarc J. Clinical use of the Kessler psychological distress scales with culturally diverse groups. Int J Methods Psychiatr Res. 2014;23(2):161–83. doi: 10.1002/mpr.1426 [published online first: 2014/04/16]

32. Cohen S, Kamarck T, Mermelstein R. A global measure of perceived stress. J Health Soc Behav. 1983;24(4):385–96. doi: 10.2307/2136404

33. Lee E-H. Review of the psychometric evidence of the perceived stress scale. Asian Nurs Res. 2012;6(4):121–27. https://doi.org/10.1016/j.anr.2012.08.004

34. Lovibond S, Lovibond P. Manual for the depression anxiety stress scales. Sydney: Psychology Foundation of Australia; 1995.

35. Henry JD, Crawford JR. The short-form version of the Depression Anxiety Stress Scales (DASS-21): construct validity and normative data in a large non-clinical sample. Br J Clin Psychol. 2005;44(Pt 2):227–39. doi: 10.1348/014466505x29657 [published online first: 2005/07/12]

36. Löwe B, Wahl I, Rose M, et al. A 4-item measure of depression and anxiety: validation and standardization of the Patient Health Questionnaire-4 (PHQ-4) in the general population. J Affect Disord. 2010;122(1–2):86–95. doi: 10.1016/j.jad.2009.06.019 [published online first: 2009/07/21]

37. Means-Christensen AJ, Arnau RC, Tonidandel AM, et al. An efficient method of identifying major depression and panic disorder in primary care. J Behav Med. 2005;28(6):565–72. doi: 10.1007/s10865-005-9023-6

38. Henkel V, Mergl R, Kohnen R, et al. Identifying depression in primary care: a comparison of different methods in a prospective cohort study. BMJ. 2003;326(7382):200–1. doi: 10.1136/bmj.326.7382.200 [published online first: 2003/01/25]

39. Jefford M, Mileshkin L, Richards K, et al. Rapid screening for depression–validation of the brief case-find for depression (BCD) in medical oncology and palliative care patients. Br J Cancer. 2004;91(5):900–6. doi: 10.1038/sj.bjc.6602057 [published online first: 2004/08/12]

CHAPTER 4

Depression and anxiety in primary care in Africa

DOI: 10.1201/9781003391531-4

4.1 DEPRESSION AND ANXIETY IN ETHIOPIA

Dawit Wondimagegn

Common mental disorders affect over 10% of the population in Ethiopia, with estimates of 12–17%, depending on the study.[1–8] The risk of developing an affective disorder (including mood and anxiety symptoms) is said to be higher among women, those with lower educational attainment and the unemployed, whereas age, marital status and ethnicity have not been found to be risk factors.[2–5]

In Ethiopia, 'illness' in general is understood to be physical; therefore, depression and anxiety do not present with 'classic' signs and symptoms.[9] This presents a significant challenge in making a diagnosis. Most patients with common mental disorders present to primary care with somatic symptoms. Medically unexplained physical symptoms involving multiple organ symptoms is the most common manifestation of mental illness across the tiers of care. Patients do not spontaneously identify their problems as being related to a mental illness.[10]

The diagnoses of depression and anxiety may not be helpful, as they are invariably associated with a fear of stigma and discrimination. This results in an immediate rejection of the diagnosis and eliminates the potential for treatment. In addition, most primary care workers are not adequately trained in the basics of clinical care and lack common skills of clinical communication and building a therapeutic alliance. This further complicates the diagnosis of mental illness in primary care settings. Instead, an approach that emphasises the relationship of physical symptoms with psychosocial stressors without going in to the details of diagnosis will encourage treatment engagement and the building of a trustful therapeutic alliance. This could later be used to make diagnosis and treatment recommendations for which the patient will then be amenable.

Depression and anxiety are not routinely diagnosed in primary care settings in Ethiopia. There are several reasons for this. The first is that most primary care workers are under-trained, over-worked and unsupported. This has created the notion that doing mental health is an additional burden on time for which there is no additional incentive. The second reason is since patients visit primary care facilities for 'physical illness' only, the opportunity for a spontaneous presentation with symptoms suggestive of a mental illness is absent. Third, even though mental health is integrated into primary care in principle, in practice, the necessary conditions are not in place to facilitate the work. Fourth, after a diagnosis is made, there are not enough and sustainable treatment options available. Finally, the lack of clear understanding of what is meant by integration and decentralisation of mental health services has led to the placement of 'mental health professionals' at primary care centres which has created role confusion. Primary care workers assume mental health work is reserved only for the mental health professionals.

There are no specific screening tools used to make a diagnosis of depression and anxiety as part of routine care. The use of screening tools is largely reserved for research purposes. There are not also other measures of distress used in primary care. Most screening and diagnosis are done through clinical interviews, and the primary care worker is expected to use clinical judgment to make a diagnosis.

Once a diagnosis of depression and/or anxiety is made, the first line of treatment is pharmacotherapy. The most commonly used antidepressant medications in Ethiopia are the class of tricyclic antidepressants (TCAs). Of these, amitriptyline is commonly used to treat depression. Most patients will be started on 25 mg, and very rarely will a primary care worker increase the dose higher enough to reach therapeutic effect. As a result, most patients on amitriptyline are under-treated, as the therapeutic dose for depression is 75 mg and above. The other available antidepressant and anti-anxiety medications are the selective serotonin reuptake inhibitors (SSRIs) fluoxetine and sertraline. Even though these medications are effective, their availability is limited. Despite attempts to introduce non-pharmaceutical psychosocial interventions through various research and implementation projects, there are no formal non-pharmaceutical interventions in primary care in Ethiopia.

A formal stepped approach to care is not part of the primary care model. However, in primary care centres where there are mid-level mental health professionals such as psychiatric nurses, a natural referral between primary care workers and the mental health professional is inevitable. This practice is not formal, and in most circumstances, primary care workers refer patients whom they suspect to have a mental illness to mental health professionals.

The detection and management of depression and anxiety in primary care in Ethiopia is not given a priority in practice. While the integration of mental health into primary care is an integral part of health policy in Ethiopia, there is a long way to go to realise this policy commitment. The pace with which this is implemented is very slow, and in most circumstances, the necessary funding and resources do not follow the policy commitment. This has rendered the primary care space into a good research platform, without leading to changes in the way things are done.

Mental health training is mainstreamed in all primary care training programmes across all universities in Ethiopia. All nursing training programmes have a mandatory course in mental health with a practicum. They cover the diagnosis and treatment of common disorders that are believed to be common in primary care. Likewise, all training programmes for doctors have mandatory training in mental health, and in some schools, this includes an internship. However, the time allotted to give these courses is invariably small in duration and is not accompanied by skills development. As a result, most graduates do not have the necessary knowledge, skill and attitude to detect and treat mental illnesses with confidence.

The detection and management of depression and anxiety in primary care in Ethiopia needs to be improved. There are several ways this could be done. To begin with, a contextual assessment of primary care workers regarding their general clinical skills that include clinical communication and therapeutic alliance needs to be conducted. To make a diagnosis of depression and anxiety, one needs to learn and be skilful in how to talk to patients. The use of screening tools in the absence of such basic clinical skills is futile. Once this assessment is done, a tailored training programme in the form of a continuing professional development could be sanctioned nationally.

Second, sustained advocacy to follow policy commitments to integrate mental health into primary care in practice, by providing the provisions necessary for primary care workers to do the job, is of paramount importance. Availability of resources is a bottleneck for improvement. Third, the development of a national framework that clearly stipulates the scope and relationships of the various actors and providers for mental health care needs to be formulated and operationalised. This will eliminate the role confusions and redundancies that hinder the provision of care. Finally, as Ethiopia has many social and traditional institutions that are engaged in the delivery of community-based, non-formal care, a platform for integration with these institutions will expand both the reach of and resources for mental health care.

REFERENCES

1. Kortmann F, Ten Horn S. Comprehension and motivation in responses to a psychiatric screening instrument validity of the SRQ in Ethiopia. Br J Psychiatry. 1988;1:95–101.
2. Mulatu MS. Prevalence and risk factors of psychopathology in Ethiopian children. J Am Acad Child Adolesc Psychiatry. 1995;34(1):100–9.
3. Tafari S, Aboud FE, Larson CP. Determinants of mental illness in a rural Ethiopian adult population. Soc Sci Med. 1991;32(2):197–201.
4. Kebede D, Alem A, Rashid E. The prevalence and socio-demographic correlates of mental distress in Addis Ababa, Ethiopia. Acta Psychiatr Scand. 1999;10:5–10.
5. Alem A, Kebede D, Woldesemiat G, Jacobsson L, Kullgren G. The prevalence and socio-demographic correlates of mental distress in Butajira, Ethiopia. Acta Psychiatr Scand. 1999;100:48–55.
6. Tadesse B, Kebede D, Tegegne T, Alem A. Childhood behavioural disorders in Ambo district, western Ethiopia. I prevalence estimates. Acta Psychiatr Scand. 1999;397:92–7.
7. Hanlon C, Medhin G, Alem A, Tesfaye F, Lakew Z, Worku B, Dewey M, Araya M, Abdulahi A, Hughes M, et al. Impact of antenatal common mental disorders upon perinatal outcomes in Ethiopia: the P-MaMiE population-based cohort study. Tropical Med Int Health. 2009;14(2):156–66.
8. Hanlon C, Medhin G, Alem A, Araya M, Abdulahi A, Tomlinson M, Hughes M, Patel V, Dewey M, Prince M. Sociocultural practices in Ethiopia: association with onset and persistence of postnatal common mental disorders. Br J Psychiatry. 2010;197(6):468–475.
9. Patel V. Explanatory models of mental illness in sub-Saharan Africa. Soc Sci Med. 1005;40(9):1291–1298.
10. Kirmayer LJ. Cultural variations in the clinical presentation of depression and anxiety: implications for diagnosis and treatment. J Clin Psychiatry. 2001;62:22–30.

4.2 DEPRESSION AND ANXIETY IN GHANA

Henry J. Lawson

The prevalence of depression in Ghana ranges between 6.7% and 25.2%, with female gender an independent risk factor for developing depression.[1] Various studies have reported different risk factors. These include lack of current employment, migration and smoking. The prenatal period in women also poses as a significant risk factor.[2] The prevalence of anxiety is much higher at 53.3%, with similar risk factors to the development of depression.[2]

Patients with depression typically present with loss of interest or lack of pleasure in things previously of interest, significant weight loss or weight gain, insomnia or excessive sleeping, fatigue or loss of energy, feelings of worthlessness or excessive guilt, poor concentration, indecisiveness, multiple bodily complaints and worrying excessively. Suicidal ideas or thoughts of death and hallucinations or delusions of morbid themes occur in severe cases.[3] In children, depression may manifest as truancy or refusal to go to school, poor school performance, bedwetting in a previously 'dry' child, odd behaviour, aggression or defiance, irritability and appetite changes.

For anxiety, the most common presentations are generalised anxiety disorder and panic disorder. Additionally, muscle tension, crawling and burning sensation around the body, restlessness or feeling on edge, sweating, being easily fatigued and palpitations may also be present.[3]

Depression and anxiety are routinely detected in primary care in Ghana. Most cases are diagnosed clinically based on symptoms and signs of the conditions and also circumstantial evidence surrounding the period when the patient reported to the health care facility. Screening tools commonly used are the Patient Health Questionnaire 2 (PHQ-2), Patient Health Questionnaire 9 (PHQ-9) and Generalized Anxiety Disorder scale (GAD-7). Baseline laboratory work includes full blood count, fasting blood sugar, blood electrolytes, urea and creatinine and thyroid function tests. In anxiety, screening for phaeochromocytoma and cardiac arrhythmias are done to rule out physiological conditions.[3]

Treatment objectives are to reduce symptoms; to prevent disruption of normal life at home, work or school; and to prevent suicide. Non-pharmaceutical interventions include reassurance, relaxation methods, regular physical exercise, counselling and cognitive behavioural therapy (CBT), which are used in an escalating fashion. If the primary care practitioner is not trained to deliver CBT, the patient is referred to a psychologist.

Usual pharmaceutical interventions are fluoxetine 20 mg daily, sertraline 50 mg daily, citalopram 20 mg daily or amitriptyline 25–50 mg daily, all for at least four weeks from the onset. For anxiety, oral propranolol may be added. Non-pharmacological methods are usually applied before these pharmacological methods are introduced.

With the passing of the Mental Health Bill and the establishment of the Mental Health Authority, coupled with the introduction of National Health Insurance, mental health disorders in general are receiving quite a boost in attention in the health care delivery space in Ghana.[4] Doctors, nurses and physician assistants are all given the relevant exposure to identify and appropriately refer cases of depression. With anxiety, arriving at the final diagnosis usually requires specialist care through psychiatrists, internists and family physicians.

Increased awareness among the population to reduce stigma and provide support for mental health conditions in general is crucial.[5] Linkage with spirituality needs to be discussed and collaboration developed with leadership on both ends.[6]

REFERENCES

1. Thapa SB, Martinez P, Clausen T. Depression and its correlates in South Africa and Ghana among people aged 50 and above: findings from the WHO study on global ageing and adult health. African J Psychiatry. 2014;17(6):10–5.
2. Amu H, Osei E, Kofie P, Owusu R, Bosoka SA, Konlan KD, et al. Prevalence and predictors of depression, anxiety, and stress among adults in Ghana: a community-based cross-sectional study. PLoS One. 2021;16(10 October):1–17. http://dx.doi.org/10.1371/journal.pone.0258105
3. Ghana Ministry of Health. *Standard Treatment Guidelines*. 7th ed. Ghana Health Service. Yamens Press Ltd, Accra; 2017:2009–2015.
4. Walker GH, Osei A. Mental health law in Ghana. BJ Psych Int. 2017;14(2):38–9.
5. Barke A, Nyarko S, Klecha D. The stigma of mental illness in Southern Ghana: attitudes of the urban population and patients' views. Soc Psychiatry Psychiatr Epidemiol. 2011;46(11):1191–202.
6. Adu P, Jurcik T, Dmitry G. Mental health literacy in Ghana: implications for religiosity, education and stigmatization. Transcult Psychiatry. 2021;58(4):516–31.

4.3 DEPRESSION AND ANXIETY IN NIGERIA

Tijani Idris Ahmad Oseni

Depression and anxiety are common in Nigeria. The prevalence of depression among primary care patients is 10–20% and 5–6% in the community.[1] Among adolescents, the prevalence is between 12.6% and 20%,[2] and in older adults it is 2.7–53.1%, while that of anxiety is 1.2–27.7%.[3] The prevalence of comorbid depression and anxiety (depression coexisting with anxiety) in Nigeria ranges from 4.3% to 20.5%.[3,4]

Patients with depression and anxiety commonly present first to their primary care provider, either at the primary health centres where they are attended to by primary care nurses, community health officers and community health extension workers, or to the general outpatient clinics of secondary and tertiary health facilities, where they are attended to by general medical practitioners and family physicians, respectively.

Patients with depression usually present with symptoms of loss of interest in previously enjoyed activities, sadness, feelings of hopelessness and impending doom, insomnia and suicidal ideation or/and attempt.[5] Patients with anxiety commonly present to the primary care clinics with feelings of worry, fear and anxiety.[5] The diagnosis is mainly clinical. Depression is usually diagnosed in primary care settings in Nigeria when a patient presents with depressed mood (sadness, irritability and emptiness) or loss of interest in activities for most of the day, for nearly all days, for two weeks. Anxiety, on the other hand, is diagnosed when a patient has excessive uncontrollable worries almost every day for six months.

Management of depression and anxiety in Nigeria is both pharmacological and non-pharmacological and includes use of psychoeducation and counselling on reduction of stressors and activation of social support networks, including family cohesion and support groups, psychotherapy, antidepressants and referral to the psychiatrist.[1,6] Group CBT has also been used in primary care clinics in Nigeria in the management of depression and anxiety, and it has been shown to be effective.[7] For depression and anxiety among the young, advocating more parental support as well as emotional counselling have helped in management.

For most primary care facilities with family physicians, management is step-wise, commencing with psychoeducation and counselling, then psychotherapy, including group CBT. Where these fail, medications are then used. Medications routinely used in most primary care facilities in Nigeria include SSRIs such as fluoxetine and sertraline and TCAs such as amitriptyline and imipramine. Patients who do not respond well to these, or in cases of severe depression, are referred to a psychiatrist for further evaluation and treatment.

Detection and management of depression and anxiety in primary care in Nigeria have been given due priority. This is evident in their inclusion into the postgraduate family medicine curriculum of the National Postgraduate Medical College of Nigeria and the West African College of Physicians. Training and retraining of family physicians and other primary care providers in the form of continuing professional development activities, workshops, seminars and webinars in mental health disorders, including depression and anxiety, are conducted regularly. This is important, as most patients present to their family doctor first and are afraid of stigmatisation associated with visiting a psychiatrist in Nigeria.

The capacity of primary care providers to promptly and adequately detect and treat patients with depression and anxiety needs to be strengthened. This can be achieved by training general practitioners, primary care nurses, community health officers and community health extension workers on the common symptoms and signs of depression and anxiety, as well as use of patient education and counselling in the management and when to refer. When properly applied, this will further reduce the burden of depression and anxiety in Nigeria.

REFERENCES

1. Adewuya AO, Adewumi T, Momodu O, Olibamoyo O, Adesoji O, Adegbokun A, Adeyemo S, Manuwa O, Adegbaju D. Development and feasibility assessment of a collaborative stepped care intervention for management of depression in the mental health in primary care (MeHPriC) project, Lagos, Nigeria. Psychol Med. 2019;49(13):2149–57.
2. Chibuike Chukwuere P, Jacobus Pienaar A, Sehularo LA. Psychosocial management of depression in adolescent learners: results and implications of a Nigerian study. J Psychol Africa. 2020;30(2):125–9.
3. Akinsulore A, Adeseiye OC, Oloniniyi IO, Esimai OA. Prevalence and factors associated with comorbid depression and anxiety among older adults in South-Western Nigeria: a community-based study. Ann Health Res. 2020 Nov 25;6(4):421–31.
4. Igbokwe CC, Ejeh VJ, Agbaje OS, Umoke PI, Iweama CN, Ozoemena EL. Prevalence of loneliness and association with depressive and anxiety symptoms among retirees in Northcentral Nigeria: a cross-sectional study. BMC Geriatr. 2020 Dec;20(1):153.
5. Ayandele O, Popoola OA, Oladiji TO. Addictive use of smartphone, depression and anxiety among female undergraduates in Nigeria: a cross-sectional study. J Health Res. 2020;34(5):443–53.
6. Gureje O, Oladeji BD, Montgomery AA, Bello T, Kola L, Ojagbemi A, Chisholm D, Araya R. Effect of a stepped-care intervention delivered by lay health workers on major depressive disorder among primary care patients in Nigeria (STEPCARE): a cluster-randomised controlled trial. Lancet Glob Health. 2019;7(7):e951–60.
7. Onyedibe MC, Nkechi AC, Ifeagwazi CM. Effectiveness of group cognitive behavioural therapy on anxiety and depression for Nigerian breast cancer patients. Int J Psychol Psychol Ther. 2020;20(2):223–32.

4.4 DEPRESSION AND ANXIETY IN SOUTH AFRICA

Bob Mash and Vanessa Lomas-Marais

In South Africa, the lifetime adult prevalence of major depressive disorders is 9.8% (standard error [SE] 0.7) and the 12-month prevalence is 4.9% (SE 0.4).[1] Of those who develop major depression, 34.3% are severe, 45.4% moderate and 20.3% mild. The differences between age groups were borderline significant ($p = 0.052$) with the highest lifetime prevalence in the 35- to 49-year age group (11.9%) and the lowest in older adults ($\geq$65 years) (6.5%).

The lifetime adult prevalence of any anxiety disorder is 15.8% (SE 0.8) with no significant differences between age groups.[1,5] For specific anxiety disorders, the lifetime prevalence is 9.8% for agoraphobia without panic, 2.7% for generalized anxiety disorder, 2.3% for post-traumatic stress disorder and 1.2% for panic disorder. The 12-month prevalence of any anxiety disorder is 8.1% (SE 0.5), and within this group 30.5% are severe, 34.4% moderate and 35.1% mild.

In terms of common mental disorders (including depression and anxiety disorders), more vulnerable demographic groups are those aged 35–49 years; those with a lower-than-average income; and those who were separated, widowed or divorced.[1] In terms of severity, vulnerable groups are women, as well as those separated, widowed or divorced.

Many ethnic groups in South Africa do not have words for depression or anxiety disorder or may describe their symptoms in such a way that they are not easily recognised. For example, in isiXhosa there is no word for depression, and phrases such as "intliziyo yam ibetha kancinci" (my heart is beating softly) may imply anxiety, but could be mistranslated as chest pain.[2] Many people with mental health problems will consult a traditional healer rather than an allopathic medical practitioner.[3]

In primary care practice, such disorders frequently present with physical symptoms.[3] In particular, different pain symptoms are common such as headache or general body pains. Comorbidity is also common, for example, with HIV, tuberculosis (TB) or diabetes. Nevertheless, if a practitioner looks for the typical symptoms of depression and anxiety, they can be identified.

A morbidity survey of primary care in the public sector found no mental health disorders in the top 25 diagnoses.[4] Schizophrenia was the most common disorder diagnosed in primary care (0.3% of consultations), only 0.2% of consultations had a diagnosis of depression and 0.1% of anxiety.[4] Depression and anxiety are therefore not routinely detected.

Primary care providers use the adult primary care (APC) guideline that integrates assessment of common symptoms with management of conditions.[5] Most consultations in public-sector primary care are with a nurse practitioner.[4] The APC links common symptoms such as fatigue, tiredness, sleeping difficulty, body pain, dizziness or breathing difficulty to the possibility of a mental disorder, such as depression or anxiety. The assessment of these conditions is linked to guidance on diagnosis (Figure 4.1). The *South African Family Practice Manual* also offers screening tools for the recognition of mental health problems and consideration of depression and anxiety.[6] However, screening tools are not routinely used in primary care.

A high workload, combined with a scarcity of well-trained practitioners in primary care (0.05 family physicians per 10,000 population in public sector[7]), means that practitioners focus on "getting through the queue". Anything that adds more time to the encounter is avoided, and this includes exploration of psychosocial and mental problems. Consultations are brief and biomedical with few person-centred communication skills.[8] Language barriers are an additional problem to making a diagnosis.[9] Most primary care providers have no or limited training in medical generalism and whole-person medicine.[10]

The South African Standard Treatment Guidelines and Essential Medicines List for Primary Care define how management is meant to happen and what medication is available.[11] The APC offers the most practical step-by-step approach to diagnosis and management for primary care providers, with a focus on the management of depression in combination with generalized anxiety disorder (Figure 4.2).[5] The primary care provider is recommended to "refer the patient for counselling and to a social worker and/or a helpline or support group". In South Africa, depression and anxiety are frequently linked to problems of living, such as poverty, unemployment, food insecurity and violence – hence the recommendation for social worker input. Professional counselling is not easily available. Few primary care facilities have a psychologist, and only the larger facilities have a social worker. More recently a new cadre of health care worker, called a registered counsellor, has been introduced, but the numbers are still small. If a counsellor is available, it is likely to be a lay counsellor with limited training and experience. Many of the larger facilities do have a nurse trained in mental health care who runs a psychiatric clinic for the cohort of patients with psychosis or severe mental health disorders that are discharged from hospital. Their capacity to provide counselling for common mental health disorders is limited. Effective counselling in primary care is therefore a barrier to care and a disincentive to diagnosis.

Three medications are available: Fluoxetine is the first-line treatment, and if not tolerated then citalopram is available. Amitriptyline is also available if sedation is desirable. A course of diazepam is available for short-term symptoms of anxiety. Additional medications such as venlafaxine and mirtazapine are available, if specialist prescribed.

Primary care providers are also encouraged to promote lifestyle changes for low mood, stress and anxiety. Advice may be given on sleep hygiene, relaxation, physical activity, limiting alcohol and substances and accessing social support.

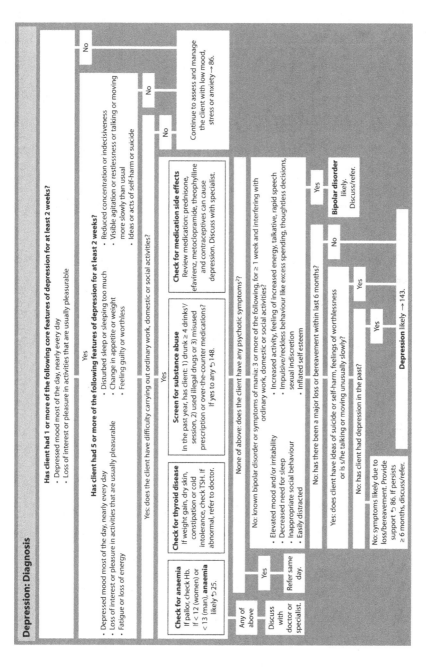

FIGURE 4.1 Diagnosis of depression in primary care in South Africa.

Depression and/or anxiety: Routine care

Assess the client with depression and/or generalised anxiety

Assess	When to assess	Note
Symptoms	Every visit	• Assess symptoms of depression and anxiety. If no better after 8 weeks of treatment or worse on treatment, discuss/refer. • Manage other symptoms as on symptom pages.
Self-harm	Every visit	Asking a client about thoughts of self-harm/suicide does not increase the chance of this. If client has suicidal thoughts or plans, refer before starting antidepressants ⤷ 83.
Mania	Every visit	If abnormally happy, energetic, talkative, irritable or reckless, discuss/refer.
Anxiety	At diagnosis	• If excessive worry causes impaired function/distress for at least 6 months with ≥ 3 of: muscle tension, restlessness, irritability, difficulty sleeping, poor concentration, tiredness: **generalised anxiety disorder** likely. • If anxiety is induced by a particular situation/object, **phobia** likely, refer/discuss. • If repeated sudden fear with physical symptoms and no obvious cause, **panic disorder** likely, refer/discuss. • If previous bad experience causing nightmares, flashbacks, avoidance of people/situations, jumpiness or a feeling of detachment, **post-traumatic stress disorder** likely ⤷ 88 and refer/discuss.
Dementia	At diagnosis	If for at least 6 months ≥ 1 of: memory problems, disorientation, language difficulty, less able to cope with daily activities and work/social function: consider **dementia** ⤷ 147.
Alcohol/drug use	Every visit	In the past year, has client:1) drunk ≥ 4 drinks/session, 2) used illegal drugs or 3) misused prescription or over-the-counter medications? If yes to any ⤷ 148.
Side effects	Every visit	Ask about side effects of antidepressant medication ⤷ 144.
Stressors	Every visit	Help identify the domestic, social and work factors contributing to depression or anxiety. If client is being abused ⤷ 88. If recently bereaved ⤷ 86.
Family planning	Every visit	• Assess client's contraceptive needs ⤷ 155. • If client pregnant or breastfeeding, doctor to discuss risks: the risk to baby from untreated depression may outweigh any risk from antidepressants. If possible, avoid antidepressants in first trimester of pregnancy. Ensure counselling/support and follow-up 2 weekly until stable. If possible, discuss with specialist.

Advise the client with depression and/or generalised anxiety

• Explain that depression is a very common illness that can happen to anybody. It does not mean that a person is lazy or weak. A person with depression cannot control his/her symptoms.
• Explain that thoughts of self-harm and suicide are common. Advise client that if s/he has these thoughts, s/he should not act, but tell a trusted person and return for help immediately.
• Educate the client that anti-depressants can take 4-6 weeks to start working. Explain that there may be some side effects, but these usually resolve in the first few days.
• Emphasise the importance of adherence even if feeling well. Advise that treatment is not addictive and not to stop treatment abruptly or without guidance.
• If difficulty with adherence, give adherence support ⤷ 170.
• Help the client to choose strategies to get help and cope:

Get enough sleep
If difficulty sleeping ⤷ 87.

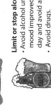

Encourage client to take time to relax:

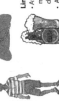

Spend time with supportive friends or family.

Find a creative or fun activity to do.

Do a relaxing breathing exercise each day.

Get active
Regular exercise might help.

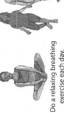

Access support
Link client with helpline or support group ⤷ 185.

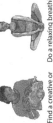

Limit or stop alcohol and avoid drugs
• Avoid alcohol until settled on medication and mood improved. Then limit alcohol to ≤ 2 drinks/day and avoid alcohol on at least 2 days/week.
• Avoid drugs.

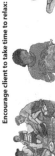

FIGURE 4.2 Adult primary care guideline in South Africa for diagnosis and management of depression and anxiety.[5]

Treat the client with depression and/or generalised anxiety

- Refer client for Counselling and to social worker and/or helpline/support group *p.185.
- Discuss benefits of antidepressants for depression and generalised anxiety disorder. Respect the client's decision if s/he declines antidepressants.
- If generalised anxiety disorder or severe anxiety¹ on starting antidepressant, consider **diazepam** 2.5–5mg daily as needed, for up to 10 days. Avoid if client is known to use substances.
- Start fluoxetine. If fluoxetine poorly tolerated, give instead citalopram. If difficulty sleeping and sedating antidepressant desired and no suicidal thoughts, start instead amitriptyline.

Medication	Dose	Note	Side effects
Fluoxetine	Start 20mg *alternate days* for 2 weeks, then increase to 20mg *daily* in the morning. If client has increased anxiety, delay increase in dose for another 2 weeks.	• Discuss with specialist if client has epilepsy, liver or kidney disease. • Monitor glucose more often in diabetes. • Advise family to monitor and return if condition worsens (suicidal thoughts or unusual changes in behaviour). • If unable to tolerate fluoxetine, stop it and start instead **citalopram** 10mg next day.	Changes in appetite and weight, headache, restlessness, difficulty sleeping, nausea, diarrhoea, sexual problems
Citalopram	Start 10mg daily for 1 week then increase to 20mg daily.	Avoid if heat failure, arrhythmias, kidney failure.	Drowsiness, difficulty, headache, dry mouth, nausea, sweating, changes in appetite and weight
Amitriptyline	Start 25mg at night. Increase by 25mg every 5 days. Review at 2 weeks: if good response, continue at this dose (75mg). If partial or no response, continue to increase by 25mg every 5 days as needed, up to 150mg/day.	Use if fluoxetine/citalopram contraindicated or poorly tolerated. Avoid if on bedaquiline, suicidal thoughts (can be fatal in overdose), heart disease, urinary retention, glaucoma, epilepsy and elderly clients.	Dry mouth, constipation, difficulty urinating, blurred vision, sedation

Decide duration of antidepressant

Has client had previous episode/s of depression and/or anxiety?

No

Does client have any of: severe depression/anxiety¹, suicidal attempt, sudden onset of symptoms, family history of bipolar disorder?

No

Does client have generalised anxiety disorder (with or without depression)?

No | Yes

Consider stopping antidepressant when client has had no/minimal symptoms and has been able to carry out routine daily activities for > 9 months.

Consider stopping antidepressant when client has had no/minimal symptoms and has been able to carry out routine daily activities for > 12 months.

Yes

Yes

Consider long term treatment for at least 3 years. If ≥ 3 episodes, advise lifelong treatment.

Reduce dose gradually over at least 4 weeks. If withdrawal occurs (irritability, dizziness, difficulty sleeping, headache, nausea, fatigue) develops, reduce even more slowly.

- Review 2 weekly, even if not on antidepressants, until symptoms get better. Then review monthly. Once stable, review 3–6 monthly.
- If no better after 8 weeks, if on antidepressant or not, refer.

FIGURE 4.2 (*Continued*)

Following the COVID-19 pandemic, there has been an increase in mental health problems. There are also major problems with substance abuse that highlight the importance of tackling mental disorders. However, the quadruple burden of disease[12] has meant that the detection and management of depression and anxiety are still lower down the list of priorities.

Doctors working in primary care are not required to have any postgraduate training in family medicine and rely on their undergraduate training in psychiatry. Such training typically focuses on severe psychiatric problems in hospital and not primary care. Nurse practitioners have only 1 year of additional training with a limited focus on mental health, often quite algorithmic in approach. Family physicians have training in mental health care (specialists in family medicine with 4 years of postgraduate training), but are limited in number and availability. There is therefore a gap in the training of primary care providers to competently detect and manage the common mental health disorders.

The detection and management of depression and anxiety in primary care need substantial improvement. We do have evidence-based guidelines and availability of essential medications. Key interventions that might improve the situation are:

- Better training of primary care providers so that they accept that this is part of their work and feel capable to detect and manage patients.
- Better availability of social services and psychological counselling in primary care.
- A model of care that reduces the workload on each provider and enables them to be more holistic in the time available.
- A model of care that provides a better skills mix in the team to diagnosis and manage patients with more complicated conditions e.g., availability of the family physician.
- A model of care that gives more priority (e.g., in monitoring and quality improvement) to common mental health disorders.

REFERENCES

1. Herman AA, Stein DJ, Seedat S, et al. The South African stress and health (SASH) study: 12-month and lifetime prevalence of common mental disorders. South African Med J. 2009;99:339–44.
2. Mash B, Mfenyana K. A different context of care. In: Mash B, ed. *Handbook of Family Medicine*. Cape Town: Oxford University Press Southern Africa, 2017:6–31.
3. Mash RJ. Are you thinking too much? Recognition of mental disorders in South African general practice. South African Fam Pract. 2000;22:22–7.
4. Mash B, Fairall L, Adejayan O, et al. A morbidity survey of South African primary care. PLoS One. 2012;7:e32358. doi:10.1371/journal.pone.0032358

5. Knowledge Translation Unit. Adult Primary Care. 2022. https://knowledgetranslation. co.za/pack/south-africa/ (accessed 3 Oct 2022).
6. Mash B. How to screen for mental problems. In: Mash B, Blitz J, eds. *South African Family Practice Manual.* Cape Town: Van Schaik, 2015:201–7.
7. Tiwari R, Mash R, Karangwa I, et al. A human resources for health analysis of registered family medicine specialists in South Africa: 2002–19. Fam Pract. 2021;38:88–94. doi:10.1093/fampra/cmaa084
8. Christoffels R, Mash B. How well do public sector primary care providers function as medical generalists in Cape Town: a descriptive survey. BMC Fam Pract. 2018;19:122. doi:10.1186/s12875-018-0802-x
9. Schlemmer A, Mash B. The effects of a language barrier in a South African district hospital. South African Med J. 2006;96:1084–7.
10. Howe A, Mash R, Hugo J. Developing generalism in the South African context. South African Med J. 2013;103:899–900.
11. National Department of Health. *Standard Treatment Guidelines and Essential Medicines List for South Africa: Primary Healthcare Level 2020 Edition.* 7th ed. Pretoria: The National Department of Health, 2020.
12. Bradshaw D, Norman R, Schneider M. A clarion call for action based on refined DALY estimates for South Africa. South African Med J. 2007;97:438–40.

CHAPTER 5

Depression and anxiety in primary care in Asia Pacific

DOI: 10.1201/9781003391531-5

5.1 DEPRESSION AND ANXIETY IN AUSTRALIA

Alison Flehr, Caroline Johnson, Catherine Kaylor-Hughes and Jane Gunn

In the 2020–2021 Australian National Survey of Mental Health and Wellbeing (NSMHWB),[1] it was estimated that 11.2% of Australians aged 16–85 (58% female) had experienced a depressive episode in their lifetime and 29% (62% female) had experienced an anxiety disorder.[2] There was also considerable overlap across the depression and anxiety groups, with around 6% of Australians reporting both.[3] The 2022 Australia's Children report ranked depression and anxiety disorders as the fifth and third leading cause of disease burden among Australian children.[4] Emerging research indicates that these rates are now likely to be higher since COVID-19.[5]

The prevalence of depression and anxiety in older Australians living in permanent residential aged care has been estimated at 46% and 15%, respectively,[6] and around 20% and 11% in Australians with a substance use disorder also experiencing depressive and anxiety disorders.[7] The mental health burden of disease for Aboriginal and Torres Strait Islander people has been estimated at 2.4 times the rate of non-indigenous Australians[8]; 30% of LGBTQIA+ Australians report a 12-month affective disorder and 45% a 12-month anxiety disorder[9]; and within an Australian transgender cohort, the prevalence of depression and anxiety was 56% and 40%, respectively.[10] Also, 58% of refugee and asylum seekers in Australia met the criteria for major depressive disorder and 60% for post-traumatic stress disorder (PTSD),[11] with cultural differences in the way mental health is perceived creating further barriers.[12]

The *Diagnostic and Statistical Manual of Mental Disorders, Fifth Edition* (DSM-V[13]) and International Statistical Classification of Diseases (ICD)-10/11[14] are routinely used in Australian primary care to define presentations that would justify a diagnosis of anxiety or depression. General practitioners (GPs) are encouraged to use the ICD-10/11 when assessing peoples' eligibility for funded mental health services.[15] However, such classifications are not always helpful in the primary care setting, as people commonly present with mixed and/or sub-threshold symptoms and require a more transdiagnostic approach.[16]

NSMHWB data showed that 20.5% of Australians with a 12-month affective disorder (61% a depressive episode)[2] and 42% of those with a 12-month anxiety disorder also reported having a physical or other long-term health condition.[17] Additionally, 49% and 57%, respectively, reported experiencing suicidal thoughts and behaviours in the last 12 months.[17] Data from a cohort of 789 patients presenting to Australian GPs with depressive symptoms found major depressive symptoms were most associated with somatic symptoms, psychiatric comorbidity, a history of childhood trauma and a long-term health problem[18]; 49% had multimorbid physical conditions, and depression prevalence increased as the number of chronic physical conditions increased.[19]

NSMHWB data also tells us that the proportion of people reporting depressive and anxiety disorders correlates with socioeconomic disadvantage.[20] Such Australians are more likely to be unemployed, not studying, receiving benefits, never married and experienced homelessness at some time in their life. Those with affective disorders were more likely to be living alone or in a non-family household, and those with anxiety disorders were more likely to be in a single-parent household.[20] Unsurprisingly, these characteristics are consistent with those flagged as 'at risk' in the Royal Australian College of General Practitioner (RACGP) Red Book preventative care guidelines.[21]

Of the 17.5% of Australians who saw a health professional for their mental health in 2020–2021, 74% saw a GP.[22] To aid in case-finding of adults requiring further assessment for depression, the RACGP Red Book recommends targeting at-risk groups and using the two-item Patient Health Questionnaire.[21] Considering anxiety disorders, no case-finding/screening tools are routinely recommended; instead, GPs identify the different anxiety disorders through consultation with their patient.[23]

To help determine the level of care the patient may need and to track depression and/or anxiety symptoms over time, Australia's Better Access initiative promotes the use of the Kessler 10 (K10) questionnaire and the Depression Anxiety Stress Scale 21 (DASS-21).[24] Importantly, while the K10 and DASS-21 can be valuable for determining symptom severity, they are not diagnostic. For the GP to make a diagnosis, they must ask questions to better understand how the patient is thinking and feeling and also consider the patient's medical history and current life events and conduct a thorough physical evaluation to properly differentiate between any mental and physical health issues.[16] GPs might also use the transdiagnostic Initial Assessment and Referral Decision Support Tool (IAR) to help assess mental health and level of care required.[25]

Currently in Australia (Figure 5.1a), in mild cases of depression and anxiety, the GP and patient will work together to identify the most pragmatic health and lifestyle modifications and self-support programmes. Ongoing care management is then left to the patient with GP support. However, most Australians presenting to primary care will have significant enough symptoms to be eligible for a Medical Benefits Scheme–funded mental health plan,[26] which is designed by the GP with the patient and features elements of goal setting, crisis planning, psychoeducation and care navigation support.[27] In cases of moderate to severe depression and/or anxiety, the mental health plan often includes specific pharmacological or psychological interventions. Between July 2020 and June 2021, Australian GPs completed over 1.5 million GP mental health treatment plans and provided over 2.4 million other mental health treatments.[28]

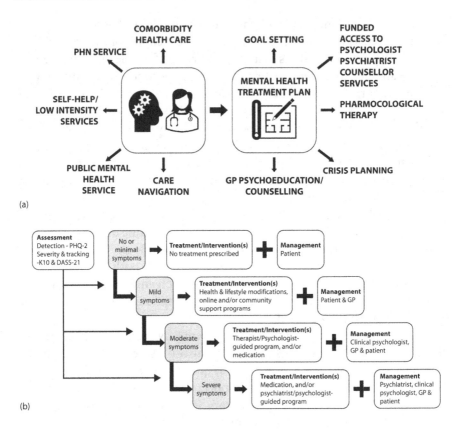

(a)

(b)

FIGURE 5.1 (a) How depression and anxiety are currently managed in Australian primary care. (b) The ambition of the Australian primary care stepped-care model. (DASS-21: Depression Anxiety and Stress Scale 21, GP: General practitioner, K10: Kessler Psychological Distress Scale, PHN: Primary health network, PHQ-2: Patient Health Questionniare-2).

GPs remain central to patients' ongoing depression and anxiety care management, and Australian primary care policy strongly supports the World Health Organization/World Organization of Family Doctors (WHO/WONCA) integrating mental health in primary care recommendations.[29] This includes the application of a patient-centred, stepped-care model (Figure 5.1b); however, due to contextual factors like workforce limitations, patient preference and communication between service and service providers,[30] this model remains something of an aspiration. Also, local experts recommend moving away from overly biomedical models in favour of more holistic approaches that are informed by people with lived experience as well as clinicians incorporating elements of social prescribing into depression and anxiety care.[31]

Since the mid-1990s, Australian health care policy makers have recognised the key role that GPs play in the detection and management of depression and anxiety. This has led to important reforms to support GPs in delivering more structured mental health care via additional training, stakeholder engagement, enhanced referral pathways and access to consultation-liaison support.[32] While these changes have facilitated help-seeking by patients, they have not always allowed for equitable access to primary care mental health services, particularly for rural and remote populations.[33] This may contribute to the high rates of antidepressant prescribing in the Australian primary care setting[34] and has led to concerted attempts to introduce stepped-care models (Figure 5.1b)[35] with the IAR as a common language between services.[36] In addition, Australian health care policy makers have recognised the value of primary care depression and anxiety research and funded high-quality studies[18] through initiatives such as Beyond Blue Victorian Centre of Excellence research grants,[37] for example.

By global standards, Australia has been an early adopter of mental e-health; for example, *MoodGYM* was one of the first internationally recognised online cognitive behavioural therapy platforms.[38] Other e-mental health tools being trialled include clinical decision support tools which aim to assist GPs in detecting depression/anxiety and making treatment recommendations,[39] for example, *StepCare*,[40] and patient-oriented care navigation support tools, such as *Link-me*.[41] Regardless, in 2020–2021 the NSMHWB estimated over 25% of Australians who consulted with a mental health professional did not have their mental health needs met.[42] In summary, Australian depression and anxiety primary care has advanced over the last 20 years, but major challenges around system navigation and integration endure[30] and shortfalls remain.

REFERENCES

1. ABS. National Study of Mental Health and Wellbeing Methodology, 2020–21 2022. Available from: https://www.abs.gov.au/methodologies/national-study-mental-health-and-wellbeing-methodology/2020-21#about-this-study accessed July 25 2022.
2. ABS. National Study of Mental Health and Wellbeing, 2020–21 2022a. Available from: https://www.abs.gov.au/statistics/health/mental-health/national-study-mental-health-and-wellbeing/2020-21/Table%202%20%E2%80%93%2012-month%20mental%20disorders.xlsx accessed July 26 2022.
3. ABS. Mental Health, 2017–18 Financial Year 2022 updated 2022/10/27/. Available from: https://www.abs.gov.au/statistics/health/mental-health/mental-health/latest-release accessed Oct 27 2022.
4. AIHW. Australia's Children, Survey Data Sources – Australian Institute of Health and Welfare 2022. Available from: https://www.aihw.gov.au/reports/children-youth/australias-children/contents/data-sources/survey-data-sources accessed Oct 28 2022.

5. AIHW. Mental Health Services in Australia, Mental Health Impact of COVID-19 – Australian Institute of Health and Welfare 2022. Available from: https://www.aihw. gov.au/getmedia/d2e9e5e2-969a-4dca-9b84-31b5fec33e46/mental-health-impact-of-covid-19.pdf.aspx accessed Oct 28 2022.

6. Amare AT, Caughey GE, Whitehead C, et al. The prevalence, trends and determinants of mental health disorders in older Australians living in permanent residential aged care: implications for policy and quality of aged care services. Aust N Z J Psychiatry. 2020;54(12):1200–11.

7. Channel BH. Substance Abuse and Mental Ilness – Dual Diagnosis 2022. Available from: https://www.betterhealth.vic.gov.au/health/conditionsandtreatments/substance-abuse-and-mental-illness-dual-diagnosis accessed Oct 27 2022.

8. AIHW. Mental Health Services in Australia: Mental Health: Prevalence and Impact 2022. Available from: https://www.aihw.gov.au/reports/mental-health-services/mental-health accessed July 26 2022.

9. ABS. National Study of Mental Health and Wellbeing, 2020–21 2022b. Available from: https://www.abs.gov.au/statistics/health/mental-health/national-study-mental-health-and-wellbeing/latest-release accessed Nov 7 2022.

10. Cheung AS, Ooi O, Leemaqz S, et al. Sociodemographic and clinical characteristics of transgender adults in Australia. Transgender Health. 2018;3(1):229–38.

11. Tay K, Frommer N, Hunter J, et al. A mixed-method study of expert psychological evidence submitted for a cohort of asylum seekers undergoing refugee status determination in Australia. Soc Sci Med. 2013;98:106–15.

12. Furler J, Kokanovic R, Dowrick C, et al. Managing depression among ethnic communities: a qualitative study. Ann Fam Med. 2010;8(3):231–36.

13. Malhi GS, Bell E, Bassett D, et al. The 2020 Royal Australian and New Zealand college of psychiatrists clinical practice guidelines for mood disorders. Aust N Z J Psychiatry. 2021;55(1):7–117.

14. AIHW. World Health Organization – Australian Institute of Health and Welfare 2020. Available from: https://www.aihw.gov.au/our-services/international-collaboration/world-health-organisation accessed Oct 31 2022.

15. RACGP. RACGP Recommendations on Mental Health Items Used in General Practice 2021 updated 2021/10/26/. Available from: https://www.racgp.org.au/FSDEDEV/media/documents/RACGP/Reports%20and%20submissions/2017/Report-RACGP-recommendations-on-Mental-Health-items-used-in-general-practice.PDF.

16. Stone L, Waldron E, Nowak H. Making a good mental health diagnosis: Science, art and ethics. Aust J Gen Pract. 2020;49(12):797–802.

17. ABS. National Study of Mental Health and Wellbeing, 2020–21 2022c. Available from: https://www.abs.gov.au/statistics/health/mental-health/national-study-mental-health-and-wellbeing/2020-21/Table%205%20%E2%80%93%2012-month%20mental%20disorders%20by%20selected%20health%20characteristics.xlsx accessed July 26 2022.

18. Gunn JM, Gilchrist GP, Chondros P, et al. Who is identified when screening for depression is undertaken in general practice? Baseline findings from the diagnosis, management and outcomes of depression in primary care (diamond) longitudinal study. Med J Aust. 2008;188:S119–S25.

19. Gunn JM, Ayton DR, Densley K, et al. The association between chronic illness, multimorbidity and depressive symptoms in an Australian primary care cohort. Soc Psychiatry Psychiatr Epidemiol. 2012;47(2):175–84.

20. ABS. National Study of Mental Health and Wellbeing, 2020–21 2022d. Available from: https://www.abs.gov.au/statistics/health/mental-health/national-study-mental-health-and-wellbeing/2020-21/Table%204%20%E2%80%93%2012-month%20mental%20disorders%20by%20population%20characteristics.xlsx accessed July 26 2022.

21. RACGP. Red Book – Guidelines for Preventative Activities in General Practice 2022. Available from: https://www.racgp.org.au/clinical-resources/clinical-guidelines/key-racgp-guidelines/view-all-racgp-guidelines/guidelines-for-preventive-activities-in-general-pr/psychosocial/introduction accessed Oct 27 2022.
22. ABS. National Study of Mental Health and Wellbeing, 2020–21 -Use of Services 2022 updated 2022/10/27/. Available from: https://www.abs.gov.au/statistics/health/mental-health/national-study-mental-health-and-wellbeing/latest-release#use-of-services accessed Oct 27 2022.
23. Kyrios M, Moulding R, Nedeljkovic M. Anxiety disorders: assessment and management in general practice. Aust Fam Physician. 2011;40(6):370–74.
24. Pirkis J, Ftanou M, Williamson M, et al. Australia's better access initiative: an evaluation. Aust N Z J Psychiatry. 2011;45(9):726–39.
25. Government A. Initial Assessment and Referral Decision Support Tool v1.05 2022. Available from: https://iar-dst.online/# accessed Oct 27 2022.
26. Australia H. Mental Health Treatment Plan 2021. Available from: https://www.healthdirect.gov.au/mental-health-treatment-plan accessed Sept 27 2022.
27. DoHA. Note AN.0.56 | Medicare Benefits Schedule: Department of Health and Ageing 2022. Available from: http://www9.health.gov.au/mbs/fullDisplay.cfm?type=note&qt=NoteID&q=AN.0.56 accessed Nov 1 2022.
28. AIHW. Mental Health Services in Australia, Medicare-Subsidised Mental Health-Specific Services – Australian Institute of Health and Welfare 2022.
29. World Health Organization, World Organization of National Colleges, Academies, and Academic Associations of General Practitioners/Family Physicians. Integrating mental health into primary care: a global perspective. World Health Organization 2008.
30. Guidelines C. Barriers to Effective Coordinated Care 2022. Available from: https://comorbidityguidelines.org.au/b4-care-coordination/barriers-to-effective-coordinated-care accessed Sept 29 2022.
31. Palmer V, Gunn J, Kokanovic R, et al. Diverse voices, simple desires: a conceptual design for primary care to respond to depression and related disorders. Fam Pract. 2010;27(4):447–58.
32. GPMHSC. General Practice Mental Health Standards Collaboration 2022. Available from: https://gpmhsc.org.au accessed Sept 28 2022.
33. Meadows GN, Enticott JC, Inder B, et al. Better access to mental health care and the failure of the Medicare principle of universality. Med J Aust. 2015;202(4):190–94.
34. Ambresin G, Palmer V, Densley K, et al. What factors influence long-term antidepressant use in primary care? Findings from the Australian diamond cohort study. Journal of Affective Disorders. 2015;176:125–32.
35. RACGP. RACGP – Mental Health Care in General Practice 2022. Available from: https://www.racgp.org.au/advocacy/position-statements/view-all-position-statements/clinical-and-practice-management/mental-health-care-in-general-practice accessed Nov 1 2022.
36. DoHA. Primary Health Networks (PHN) Mental Health Care Guidance – Initial Assessment and Referral for Mental Health Care 2022.
37. BeyondBlue. Beyond Blue 2022. Available from: https://www.beyondblue.org.au/about-us/who-we-are-and-what-we-do/20-years-of-beyond-blue accessed Nov 28 2022.
38. Twomey C, O'Reilly G. Effectiveness of a freely available computerised cognitive behavioural therapy programme (MoodGYM) for depression: meta-analysis. Aust N Z J Psychiatry. 2017;51(3):260–69.

39. Fletcher S, Chondros P, Densley K, et al. Matching depression management to severity prognosis in primary care: results of the target-D randomised controlled trial. Br J Gen Pract. 2021;71(703):e85–e94.

40. Whitton AE, Hardy R, Cope K, et al. Mental health screening in general practices as a means for enhancing uptake of digital mental health interventions: observational cohort study. J Med Internet Res. 2021;23(9):e28369.

41. Fletcher S, Spittal MJ, Chondros P, et al. Clinical efficacy of a decision support tool (Link-me) to guide intensity of mental health care in primary practice: a pragmatic stratified randomised controlled trial. Lancet Psychiatry. 2021;8(3):202–14.

42. ABS. National Study of Mental Health and Wellbeing, 2020–21 2022e. Available from: https://www.abs.gov.au/statistics/health/mental-health/national-study-mental-health-and-wellbeing/2020-21/Table%207%20%E2%80%93%20Perceived%20need%20for%20 help%20for%20people%20who%20consulted%20a%20health%20professional.xlsx accessed Sept 28 2022.

5.2 DEPRESSION AND ANXIETY IN HONG KONG, SAR

Amy Pui Pui Ng, Weng Yee Chin and Julie Yun Chen

The prevalence of common mental disorders (depression and/or anxiety) is 13.3% in the Hong Kong (HK) general population.[1] Mixed anxiety and depression disorder and general anxiety disorder account for 6.9% and 4.2%, respectively.[1] A reported 10.7% of patients in HK primary care clinics screen positive for depression.[2] Research in HK shows that common mental disorders are associated with being female, being divorced or separated, misusing alcohol or substances, lacking regular exercise and having a family history of mental disorders.[1] At-risk populations for depression include patients who are unemployed, have a past history of depression, are female, are aged 35 years or older, have no regular exercise, have a family history of mental health problems or are not ethnically Chinese.[2]

Twenty-six per cent of patients in HK with common mental disorders have consulted a health professional for their mental health problem in the past year.[1] Similarly, 23% of patients who screened positive in primary care clinics for depression received a diagnosis of depression by the doctor.[2] Other studies show that only between 3.5% and 9% of patients with a depressive episode, general anxiety disorder, mixed anxiety and depression disorder and other anxiety disorder had consulted primary care physicians (PCPs) for their mental health problems in the past year.[1] Despite low detection rates of mental disorders and presence of screening instruments such as PHQ-9 and GAD-7, which have been validated and demonstrated to be sensitive screening instruments among Chinese patients in primary care settings,[3] there is currently no recent local primary care guideline advocating their use for screening and detection. Only 6–8% of PCPs use screening instruments and 42–72% use the DSM or ICD criteria for diagnosis, with 26–48% claiming to have no specific criteria for diagnosis.[4]

Without locally produced guidelines, most PCPs in HK follow international guidelines such as National Institute for Health and Care Excellence (NICE),[5,6] and thus, treatments are based on the severity of the symptoms. For mild symptoms, patients are managed by their usual PCP conservatively by providing metal health education, psychological support and behavioural advice. Due to the high cost of private specialist psychiatric services, and despite long waiting times, most patients (70%) choose government psychiatric services if a psychiatric referral is necessary.[7] One option is the Hospital Authority's Integrated Mental Health Program (IMHP) launched in 2010, which is based on a family doctor–led collaborative care model[8,9] and delivered in the public primary care setting. The IMHP uses the PHQ-9 and GAD-7 for screening, risk stratification and monitoring and uses a stepped-care approach for patient management.[10] Apart from being managed by their usual PCP, patients with mild symptoms can enrol in group-based empower-ment courses. For moderate symptoms, patients can be referred to the IMHP, where key workers (nurses, occupational therapists and social workers) con-duct further assessments and provide non-drug interventions such as behav-ioural activation and problem-solving treatment. Key workers will alert the PCP for cases at high risk for deterioration or non-response. For those with severe symptoms or requiring drug treatments, key workers and IMHP doc-tors will manage the patient collaboratively. IMHP doctors have higher family medicine qualifications than most PCPs working in general outpatient clin-ics. IMHP patients with suicidal risk or psychotic symptoms are referred to the emergency department or psychiatrist. IMHP doctors regularly meet with psychiatrists and key workers to discuss severe/difficult cases.[10]

A territory-wide observational study conducted in 2015 found in patients diagnosed with depressive symptoms by their PCP, 51% were prescribed med-ications, of whom 84% were prescribed antidepressants, 41% were provided counselling and 39% were referred to other health care providers.[2] Another study found that in those with general anxiety disorder, only 4.1% received selective serotonin reuptake inhibitors, and a majority of patients receiving tranquillizers and hypnotics were unaware of the risk of dependence or no treatment.[11]

The Hospital Authority, the body that runs all public hospitals and clin-ics, published a Mental Health Service Plan 2010–2015 which stressed the importance of primary care in diagnosing and managing common mental disorders and led to the implementation of the IMHP in 2010. IMHP has five objectives: Early identification and intervention of those with common mental disorders, avoiding stigmatisation by managing these patients in the community, empowering primary care clinics to manage common mental disorders, reducing psychiatric referrals and improving the quality of pri-mary health care in whole-person management.[10] However, three-quarters of patients still do not seek mental health support by health professionals or receive a diagnosis of a mental health problem despite the need.[1,2] From the patient's perspective, barriers to seeking professional help in HK include wor-ries about drug side effects (80%) and drug dependency (75%), affordability of medical fees (71%) and reluctance to be referred to a psychiatrist.[7,12] Also, over one-third of patients agreed that psychological distress could get better without professional help.[13] From the health provider's perspective, PCPs in HK feel that the major barrier to managing mental health disorders is because it is too time-consuming (81%), there is a lack of supporting services (29%) including lack of timely access to public psychiatrists and lack of feedback from psychiatrists after referrals and lack of experience (20.2%).[12,14] Doctors in HK are not required to have vocational training to practice in primary care. Becoming a specialist in family medicine requires completing six years of training and examination. Research shows that doctors with higher qualifications in family medicine are more confident in managing mental health patients, use more standardised criteria for diagnosis and use more psychotherapy compared with those without.[4,14]

Therefore, increasing the training of PCPs on common mental health disorders is crucial. The development of national guidelines may help to standardise care and encourage more consistent screening and management by PCPs. To address the "too time-consuming" barrier, having alternative forms of remuneration for treating these disorders will help doctors feel it is worthwhile to see such patients,[14] or in the public sector, having a designated protected time to see such patients may help. From the perspective of primary prevention, mental health policy should target screening for at-risk groups such as females, divorced or separated individuals and those with a personal or family history of mental health problems. Training of other primary care personnel and promotion of all citizens having a family doctor may improve the detection rates and management of mental health problems.

REFERENCES

1. Lam LC-W, Wong CS-M, Wang M-J, Chan W-C, Chen EY-H, Ng RM-K, et al. Prevalence, psychosocial correlates and service utilization of depressive and anxiety disorders in Hong Kong: the Hong Kong Mental Morbidity Survey (HKMMS). Soc Psychiatry Psychiatr Epidemiol. 2015;50(9):1379–88.
2. Chin WY, Chan KTY, Lam CLK, Wong SYS, Fong DYT, Lo YYC, et al. Detection and management of depression in adult primary care patients in Hong Kong: a cross-sectional survey conducted by a primary care practice-based research network. BMC Fam Pract. 2014;15(1):30.
3. Chiu B, Chin W. Systematic review and meta-analysis on the patient health questionnaire-9 (PHQ-9) for depression screening in Chinese primary care patients. Family Med Care. 2018;1(1):1–2.
4. Wong S, Lee K, Chan K, Lee A. General practitioners with a higher qualification in family medicine or general practice: are they better in diagnosing and treating patients with depression and anxiety? Hong Kong Pract. 2007;29(9):348.
5. Wong SY, Tang W, Mak WW, Cheung F, Mercer S, Griffiths S, et al. Stepped care programme in primary care to prevent anxiety and depression: a randomised clinical trial. Hong Kong Med J. 2019;25(suppl 3):9–10.
6. Wong MM. Update on the management of depressive disorder in primary care settings. Hong Kong Pract. 2014;36:12–9.
7. Sun KS, Lam TP, Lam KF, Lo TL, Chao DVK, Lam EWW. Barriers of Chinese primary care attenders to seeking help for psychological distress in Hong Kong. J Affect Disord. 2016;196:164–70.
8. Unützer J, Park M. Strategies to improve the management of depression in primary care. Prim Care: Clinics in Office Practice. 2012;39(2):415–31.
9. Goodrich DE, Kilbourne AM, Nord KM, Bauer MS. Mental health collaborative care and its role in primary care settings. Curr Psychiatry Rep. 2013;15(8):383.
10. Chu D. Integrated Mental Health Programme Common Mental Disorder patients in GOPC Hong Kong: Hospital Authority. 2014. Available from: https://www3.ha.org.hk/haconvention/hac2014/proceedings/downloads/MC2.3.pdf.

11. Lee S, Tsang A, Chui H, Kwok K, Cheung E. A community epidemiological survey of generalized anxiety disorder in Hong Kong. Community Ment Health J. 2007;43(4):305–19.
12. Sun KS, Lam TP, Lam KF, Lo TL. Obstacles in managing mental health problems for primary care physicians in Hong Kong. Adm Policy Ment Health. 2015;42(6):714–22.
13. Sun KS, Lam TP, Lam KF, Lo TL, Chao DVK, Lam EWW, et al. Views of Hong Kong Chinese primary care attenders on psychological distress: causes, management and recovery. Fam Pract. 2019;36(1):84–90.
14. Wong SYS, Lee K, Chan K, Lee A. What are the barriers faced by general practitioners in treating depression and anxiety in Hong Kong? Int J Clin Pract. 2006;60(4):437–41.

5.3 DEPRESSION AND ANXIETY IN MALAYSIA

Sherina Mohd Sidik, Noor Ani Ahmad and Nurashikin Ibrahim

In 2015 the Malaysian National Health and Morbidity Survey (NHMS) estimated that 29.9% of adults in Malaysia were experiencing mental health problems such as depression and anxiety, obtained using the General Health Questionnaire (GHQ-12). This number represented a three-fold increase from the prevalence of 10.7% estimated by the NHMS in 1996.[1] In 2019, NHMS yielded a 2.3% prevalence of depression among Malaysians 18 years old and above, using the Patient Health Questionnaire (PHQ-9).[2] The specific at-risk populations were the elderly, single, widowed, low socioeconomic status and females.[1,2]

Depression and anxiety are routinely detected using selected validated questionnaires in Malaysian government primary care clinics. The screening tool used was the Depression, Anxiety and Stress Scale (DASS-21). Screening was implemented under the Healthy Mind Services in Primary Care with the aim to decentralise the mental health services as one of the key strategies in a primary health care shift from curative to preventive care. Additional mental health services at primary care also includes integrated mental health screening using the BSSK (Health Status Screening Form) for adolescents, adults and the elderly.[3] Patients attending government primary care clinics are screened using the selected questionnaires while in the waiting area to see the doctor. The screening and scoring are done by the nurses and medical assistants. Patients with high scores are referred to see the doctors and/ or family medicine specialists, where the final diagnosis will be made by the attending doctor depending on the patient's scores and their clinical judgement. There is a structured guideline which details how each patient is to be managed depending on their scores.

Recently the Whooley 2-Questions on Depression, GAD 2-item, the Malay-validated PHQ-9 and the Malay-validated GAD-7 were implemented to replace the DASS-21 in primary care settings in Malaysia. This is a two-phase screening process using the Whooley 2-Questions, followed by the PHQ-9 to detect depression, and the GAD-2 followed by the GAD-7 to detect anxiety, respectively, in primary care clinics.[4]

For depression, the first phase using the Whooley 2-Questions involves explaining the purpose of the screening to the patients first, and then, a time limit of 5–10 minutes is given to the patient to complete the questionnaire. The results are interpreted as either "no risk for depression," where the patient will proceed to the health education talk, which is routinely conducted in primary care clinics for all patients, or "at risk for depression" for patients who answer "Yes" to one or both of the Whooley 2-Questions, and these patients will be required to complete the PHQ-9.[4]

For the second phase of screening, the patients are also given the same time limit of 5–10 minutes to complete the PHQ-9. The total scores are calculated by the attending health personnel (either a nurse or medical assistant) and the patients informed of their total scores, what this means and how to proceed with subsequent management. For total scores 0–4 (normal), patients are given health education advice and healthy lifestyle practices. For total scores of 5–9 (mild depression), patients are referred to the medical officer for further assessment. For total scores ≥10 (moderate/severe/very severe depression) and/or "YES" for Question No. 9 of the PHQ-9 which asks about suicide risk, the patients are referred to the medical officer and subsequently to a family medicine specialist if required.[4]

There are also two phases of screening in the detection of anxiety. The first phase uses the GAD-2. Similarly, the purpose of the screening is first explained to the patients, and a time limit of 5–10 minutes is given to the patient to complete the questionnaire. The results are interpreted as either "no risk for anxiety" (total score <3) where the patient proceeds to the health education talk or "at risk for anxiety" (total score ≥3) where these patients are required to complete the GAD-7.[4]

Patients are also given the same time limit of 5–10 minutes to complete the GAD-7. For total scores 0–4 (normal), they receive the health education advice about healthy lifestyle practices. For total scores 5–9 (mild depression), patients are referred to the medical officer for further assessment. For total scores ≥10 (moderate/severe/very severe anxiety), they are referred to the medical officer and subsequently a family medicine specialist if required.[4]

For both depression (PHQ-9 scores ≥ 10) and anxiety (GAD-7 scores ≥10), diagnosed cases are registered as new cases, and an appointment date for follow-up treatment with the medical officer or family medicine specialist is given. Patients can also be referred to counsellors at the clinics. Treatment may also include medication with antidepressants such as selective serotonin reuptake inhibitors (SSRIs). For cases where the diagnosis is unclear, they will be referred to the visiting psychiatrist in some clinics. At clinics without visiting psychiatrists, these patients will be referred to psychiatrists in nearby government hospitals.[4]

The detection and management of depression and anxiety in primary care are given priority in Malaysia, where all government primary care clinics implement the screening process for depression and anxiety. Our primary care personnel (nurses, medical assistants, doctors) are trained to detect these disorders; special training is conducted for all primary care personnel selected to be in charge of the mental health screening in their clinics. In 2020, screening using Whooley-2 Questions and GAD-7 was implemented as a pilot project in six states throughout Malaysia, which were Selangor, Wilayah Persekutuan, Kuala Lumpur, Putrajaya, Negeri Sembilan and Perlis. The

Mental Health Screening and Intervention Programme in Primary Care was then further expanded to involve more primary care clinics throughout the country, and currently there are 1,161 clinics implementing this programme. In 2022, an additional 200 psychology counselling officers were placed at the district and health clinics in primary care to provide intervention and counselling services to those with mental health conditions including anxiety and depression.

To further strengthen this programme, there are plans to provide this screening to patients attending antenatal and postnatal visits at primary care clinics as well. This service can also be improved by implementing integrated care for all patients and involve multidisciplinary care that includes family members.

REFERENCES

1. Institute for Public Health National Health and Morbidity Survey 2015 (NHMS 2015). Vol. II: Non-Communicable Diseases, Risk Factors & Other Health Problems. Malaysia: Ministry of Health. 2015.
2. National Health and Morbidity Survey (NHMS) 2019 (NMRR-18-3085-44207). Non-Communicable Diseases, Healthcare Demand, and Health Literacy: Key Findings. © 2020 Institute for Public Health, National Institutes of Health, Ministry of Health Malaysia. ISBN 978-983-99320-6-5
3. National Strategic Plan for Mental Health 2020–2025. Copyright @Ministry of Health Malaysia. Mental Health, Injury Prevention and Violence and Substance Abuse Sector (MeSVIPP) Non-Communicable Disease Section Disease Control Division. ISBN 978-967-2469-21-6
4. Garis Panduan Saringan Minda Sihat di Fasiliti Kesihatan Primer Edisi 2/2021. Unit Kesihatan Mental Sektor MeSVIPP, Bahagian Kawalan Penyakit, Kementerian Kesihatan Malaysia. "Healthy Mind Screening Guidelines in Primary Health Facilities Edition 2/2021. Mental Health Unit Section MESVIPP, Disease Control Division, Ministry of Health Malaysia."

CHAPTER 6

Depression and anxiety in primary care in the East Mediterranean

DOI: 10.1201/9781003391531-6

6.1 ANXIETY AND DEPRESSION IN EGYPT

Nagwa Nashat Hegazy

Earlier surveys of psychiatric morbidity among the Egyptian population revealed that the prevalence of depression and anxiety was 15.3% and 36%, respectively.[1,2] A country-wide survey by Egypt's Ministry of Health indicated in c. 2018 that approximately 25% of Egyptians suffer from mental health issues, with about 44% of these suffering from anxiety and depression disorders.[3] These rates varied according to age and residence. Urban populations had less depression (11.4%) compared with rural populations (19.7%), and the reported prevalence of depression and anxiety in the elderly was 23.7–74.5% and 14.2–72%, respectively.[4] The reported discrepancy in the prevalence of anxiety and depression is due to varied data collection settings and inconsistency of the diagnostic tools. It was noted that residential homes and community clubs had a lower prevalence compared with inpatient and household community surveys.[4]

At-risk populations for mental disorders are usually associated with sociodemographic factors such as being female, unemployed, increasing age, divorced, non-educated or lower educational status, living alone and insufficient income and the presence of comorbidities (e.g., heart, kidney or liver disease; hypertension; diabetes mellitus; lower back pain; and pulmonary conditions).[4–6]

The profile of psychiatric presentation in Egypt reveals that individuals with anxiety may present initially with tension-related physical symptoms such as headache, a pounding heart or insomnia,[7] followed by worrying, irritability, free-floating, tiredness, restlessness and anergia.[6] Depression among Egyptian patients manifests mainly with one or more physical symptoms, such as pain or tiredness all the time,[7] or the patient can present with agitation, decreased libido, anorexia, hypochondriasis and insomnia. In Egyptian patients, affect may be masked by multiple somatic symptoms which occupy the foreground, with the affective component of their illness receding into the background.[6,8] Although these are common symptoms, anxiety and depression are often under-recognised and under-treated. These symptoms act as warning signs for family physicians to start mental health assessment and a psychiatric interview, which necessitates a trained, orientated and qualified family physician.

The new guidelines for mental health in primary care for physicians are based on guidelines from the World Health Organization (WHO).[9] Diagnosis is accomplished in four major steps: (1) Conducting a brief mental health assessment, (2) using the appropriate interactive summary card and flow chart, (3) using the Arabic Questionnaire and (4) using the symptom index and general flow charts. Conducting a brief mental health assessment is done to gather enough information. This is aimed to identify the presenting

Interactive Summary Cards and Flow Chart Assessment Guide

To be used with I C.D10 PC

Anxiety

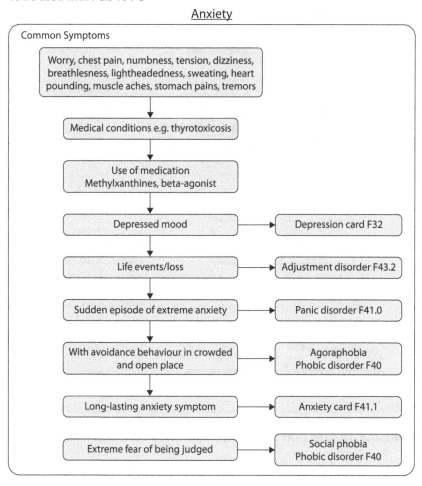

FIGURE 6.1 Anxiety interactive summary card and flow chart.

complaint and other associated features to verify the appropriate interactive summary card and flow chart to use. Depression and anxiety both have interactive summary cards and a flow chart containing the main symptoms as well as the overlapping ones (see Figures 6.1 and 6.2).[7]

The Arabic Questionnaire is then used to confirm the provisional diagnosis. It can be completed by patients during the consultation or after their first visit, either alone or with the help of an assistant. The Symptom Index and the general flow charts help to identify the severity of the disorder and assist general practitioners in their everyday decision-making.[7]

Flow Chart Assessment Guide to Be Used with I.C.D10 PC Depression

Common symptoms

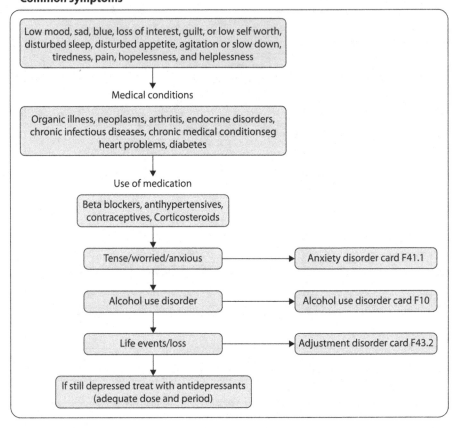

FIGURE 6.2 Depression interactive summary card and flow chart.

Several psychotherapeutic strategies have been suggested to overcome anxiety and depression, and pharmacotherapeutic augmentation treatment is the recommended second choice in cases where there is insufficient response to the initial management.[8] Anxiety and depression treatment begins with patient and family counselling and support. The patient is encouraged to engage in physical activities and is taught structured problem-solving techniques. If significant anxiety symptoms persist despite the suggested measures, *Valeriana* root capsule or antidepressant drugs such as imipramine can be used. Adding beta-blockers may help to control physical symptoms such as tremor. In cases of depression, the choice of medication is tailored to the patient's condition provided there is an absence of red flags and the drug is included in the essential psychotropic medication list.[7]

In anxiety, non-urgent referral is advised if the patient's symptoms are severe or affecting social or occupational functioning. Referral to secondary mental health services in depression is advised in an emergency, if there is a significant risk of suicide or danger to others, psychotic symptoms or severe agitation. Non-emergency referral is indicated in case of medical treatment failure.[7]

Mental health services in primary care in Egypt have only been established recently. As these services were mainly provided by hospitals, insufficient attention was given to integration of mental health into primary care. National mental health programmes were instigated in 1991–1996 and in 1997–2003 to include mental health in primary health care.[8] However, this strategy failed to gain acceptance because it did not address the lack of public awareness of mental health issues, the stigma associated with mental illness or, most importantly, the need to shift psychiatric care from asylums to the community. In 2006, a public awareness project was started to address this, and it has been taken as a priority since then.[10]

Changing clinical practices and public attitudes is a lengthy process, and Egypt is witnessing the very beginning of this change. Implementation so far has been limited. The infrastructure and services are grossly insufficient for the large and growing needs. Cultural beliefs affect interpretation of mental symptoms. Integration of mental health into primary care started in five governorates, and training was conducted with follow-up, supervision and a referral system to secondary care in order to support primary care physicians. To date the programme has trained 642 physicians, 959 nurses and 468 social workers and health educators in 300 primary health care units.[9]

REFERENCES

1. Okasha A. Prevalence of depressive disorders in a sample of rural and urban Egyptian communities. Egypt J Psychiatry. 1988;11:167–81.
2. Okasha A, Kamel M, Sadek A, Lotaif F, Bishry Z. Psychiatric morbidity among university students in Egypt. Br J Psychiatry. 1977;131(2):149–54.
3. Egypt Today Staff. 25% of Egyptians Suffer from Mental Health Issues: Survey. Egypt Today. April 18 2018. Available from: https://www.egypttoday.com/Article/1/48156/25-of-Egyptians-suffer-from-mental-health-issues-survey accessed Oct 23 2022.
4. Odejimi O, Tadros G, Sabry N. A systematic review of the prevalence of mental and neurocognitive disorders amongst older adults' populace in Egypt. Middle East Curr Psychiatry. 2020;27(1):1–2.
5. Ahmed D, Shair E, Taher IH, Zyada E. F. Prevalence and predictors of depression and anxiety among the elderly population living in geriatric homes in Cairo. Egypt J Egypt Public Health Assoc. 2014;89(3):127–35.
6. Ghanem M, Gadallah M, Meky FA, Mourad S, El Kholy G. (2009). National survey of prevalence of mental disorders in Egypt: preliminary survey. East Mediterr Health J. 2009;15(1):65–75.
7. Mental Health In. Abdel Megid S (ed.). Practice Guidelines for Family Physicians. Volume 5. 3rd edition. Egypt;2018, pp. 57–103.

8. Okasha A. Focus on psychiatry in Egypt. Bri J Psychiatry. 2004;185(3):266–72.
9. Jenkins R, Heshmat A, Loza N, Siekkonen I, Sorour E. Mental health policy and development in Egypt-integrating mental health into health sector reforms 2001-9. Int J Ment Health Syst. 2010 Dec;4(1):1–1.
10. Loza N. Integrating Egyptian mental health services into primary care: the policy maker's perspective. Int Psychiatry. 2010;7(1):5–6.

6.2 DEPRESSION AND ANXIETY IN TUNISIA

Malek Chaabouni and Asma Chaabouni

Prevalence rates of depression and anxiety are mainly documented in scientific studies, as there is a lack of an available data registry on psychological problems in Tunisia.[1] Estimated prevalence rates of depression and anxiety in general settings varies between 38% and 70%.[2,3] Depression and anxiety rates in specific vulnerable populations, such as victims of domestic violence or residents in medicine, are typically higher and range between 50% and 70%.[4,5] Although these studies provide evidence that anxiety and depression are highly prevalent in Tunisia, these results cannot be generalised. In fact, study populations are often small and not representative.[2-4] Additionally, these studies typically rely on self-report measures, known for over-estimating morbidity rates.[2-4,6]

As in several African countries, it is not uncommon that patients with mental health difficulties in Tunisia present with somatic symptoms.[7] This might be linked to several factors, such as a high level of stigma around mental illness and a lack of self-awareness.[8] Health care professionals find making the diagnosis of depression and anxiety when the patient presents with only somatic symptoms challenging. In the case of the absence of a somatic disease, these somatic symptoms are typically related to high levels of stress and social circumstances and rarely related to mental health problems.

Even though Tunisian family physicians (FPs) and GPs manage 30–40% of mental health problems, GPs and FPs often report being uncomfortable in managing patients with mental health difficulties.[9,10] Therefore, routine detection of depression and anxiety in primary care has yet to be improved. It is still not common to use screening tools to detect depression and anxiety in primary care. This might be due to several barriers. Firstly, even though several screening tools for depression and anxiety have been validated in Arabic, few have explicitly been developed in Tunisian dialect and taking into consideration cultural specificities.[11] Additionally, patients often seek help from their GPs and FPs at an advanced stage of their mental health problems. Because of the severity and the high number of symptoms at these stages of the disease, the diagnosis of depression or anxiety is often obvious based on medical interviews. Furthermore, GPs and FPs typically need more time in consultations for mental health problems. Therefore, screening tools might be considered time-consuming.

Around one-third of patients, who suffer from mental health problems report visiting traditional healers before seeing a mental health expert.[11]

Management of depression and anxiety in Tunisia differs between the public and the private sectors. In the public sector, a balanced care model is put into place, where GPs and FPs play the role of gatekeepers. GPs and FPs can then choose either to manage the patient in primary care or to refer them to one of the few psychiatric institutions and departments. Treatment options are mainly medication. Talking therapies such as cognitive behavioural therapy (CBT) could be offered in some cases, mainly in secondary care. In the private sector, patients have direct access to psychiatrists and mental health professionals with no need to contact their GP or FP. Treatment options for psychological problems are more diverse, including talking therapies and medication.

A great deal of attention has been recently paid to improving mental health services in primary care in Tunisia, including detection and management. As such, recent programmes have been introduced for both GPs and residents in family medicine. For GPs, a training programme launched by the WHO, entitled the Mental Health Gap Action Programme (mhGAP), was implemented in 2017 with the aim of training GPs to diagnose and treat mental health problems.[12] The outcomes after the training were promising and showed that GPs had improved their knowledge on how to deal with mental health difficulties.[12]

For residents in family medicine, a training programme in a psychiatric department has been introduced, and it is currently mandatory to validate this before being qualified to practice as an FP. The aim of this training programme is to gain autonomy in diagnosing and treating mental health problems, yet the quality of training may vary among departments and universities.

Primary care personnel do not usually have extra training to screen for these disorders. GPs and FPs could apply for diplomas hosted by their correspondent faculty of medicine to gain extra competencies. Examples are diplomas in addiction psychology and diplomas in CBT. However, these diplomas are open to all medical doctors and therefore not specific to the knowledge of a GP or FP.

The mental health sector faces several challenges, including stigma around mental health problems,[9,12–14] restrictions around prescribing psychotropic drugs in primary care,[14,15] the lack of funding to improve mental health care in primary care,[9,14] the limited number of mental health professionals, who mainly practice in the north and the centre of the country,[13,16] and the lack of training in managing mental health disorders by GPs and FPs.[16–19] One of the ways to improve the management of depression and anxiety in primary care is to create mandatory contextualised training programmes as an opportunity to enhance GPs' and FPs' confidence in engaging and managing mental health illnesses.[15]

REFERENCES

1. Charfi F, Ouali U, Spagnolo J, Belhadj A, Nacef F, Saidi O, Melki W. Highlighting successes and challenges of the mental health system in Tunisia: an overview of services, facilities, and human resources. J Ment Health. 2021;1–9. doi: 10.1080/09638237.2021.1875414.

2. Bouattour W, Turki M, Ellouze S, Messedi N, Charfeddine F, Halouani N, Aribi L, Aloulou J. Psychological responses of Tunisian general population during COVID-19 pandemic. Pan Afr Med J. 2021;40:74. doi: 10.11604/pamj.2021.40.74.26379.

3. Kharroubi G, Cherif I, Amor SH, Zribi M, Atigue WB, Ouali U, Bettaieb J. Mental health status of adults under institutional quarantine: a cross-sectional survey in Tunisia. Pan Afr Med J. 2021;40:197. doi: 10.11604/pamj.2021.40.197.31112.

4. Jbir R, Aribi L, Abid W, Jbir I, Charfeddine F, Ellouze S, Aloulou J. Anxiety and depression among Tunisian women victims of domestic violence. Eur Psychiatry. 2022;65:S318–S318. doi: 10.1192/j.eurpsy.2022.810.

5. Marzouk M, Ouanes-Besbes L, Ouanes I, Hammouda Z, Dachraoui F, Abroug F. Prevalence of anxiety and depressive symptoms among medical residents in Tunisia: a cross-sectional survey. BMJ Open. 2018;8:e020655. doi: 10.1136/bmjopen-2017-020655.

6. Kroenke K, Spitzer RL, Williams JBW, Löwe B. The patient health questionnaire somatic, anxiety, and depressive symptom scales: a systematic review. Gen Hosp Psychiatry. 2010;32:345–359. doi: 10.1016/j.genhosppsych.2010.03.006.

7. Lasater ME, Beebe M, Warren NE, Souko F, Keita M, Murray SM, Bass JK, Surkan PJ, Winch PJ. Dusukasi—The heart that cries: an idiom of mental distress among perinatal women in rural Mali. Cult Med Psychiatry. 2018;42:930–945. doi: 10.1007/s11013-018-9579-6.

8. Khiari H, Ouali U, Zgueb Y, Mrabet A, Nacef F. Pathways to mental health care for patients with severe mental illness in Tunisia. Pan Afr Med J. 2019;34:118. doi: 10.11604/pamj.2019.34.118.19661.

9. Ben Salah F. Stratégie nationale de la promotion de la santé mentale. Tunisie: Ministère de la santé unité de la santé mentale; 2013.

10. Melki M, Bouslah A, Fendri C, Mâalel I, Zâafrane F, Khiari G, Jebara H, Gaha L. Attitudes etconduites pratiques des médecins de première ligne face à la santé mentale dans la région de Monastir. Tunis; VIII Journée de la Santé Publique de Monastir. 2003.

11. Ali G-C, Ryan G, De Silva MJ. Validated screening tools for common mental disorders in low and middle income countries: a systematic review. PLoS ONE. 2016;11:e0156939. doi: 10.1371/journal.pone.0156939.

12. Spagnolo J, Champagne F, Leduc N, Melki W, Guesmi I, Bram N, Guisset A-L, Piat M, Laporta M, Charfi F. Tailoring a training based on the mental health gap action programme (mhGAP) intervention guide (IG) to Tunisia: process and relevant adaptations. Glob Ment Health (Camb). 2018;5:e17. doi: 10.1017/gmh.2018.8.

13. World Health Organization and Ministry of Health Tunisia. WHO-AIMS Report on Mental Health System in Tunisia. Tunisia. 2008.

14. Spagnolo J, Champagne F, Leduc N, Melki W, Bram N, Guesmi I, Rivard M, Bannour S, Bouabid, Ganzoui SBHH, et al. A program to further integrate mental health into primary care: lessons learned from a pilot trial in Tunisia. J Glob Health Rep. 2019;3:e2019022. doi: 10.29392/joghr.3.e2019022.

15. Spagnolo J, Champagne F, Leduc N, Melki W, Piat M, Laporta M, Bram N, Guesmi I, Charfi F. "We find what we look for, and we look for what we know": factors interacting with a mental health training program to influence its expected outcomes in Tunisia. BMC Public Health. 2018;18:1398. doi: 10.1186/s12889-018-6261-4.

16. Spagnolo J, Champagne F, Leduc N, Piat M, Melki W, Charfi F, Laporta M. Building system capacity for the integration of mental health at the level of primary care in Tunisia: a study protocol in global mental health. BMC Health Serv Res. 2017;17:38. doi: 10.1186/s12913-017-1992-y.

17. Elloumi H, Zalila H, Kallel G, Cheour, Boussetta A. Attitude des médecins généralistes face à la schizophrénie. Tunis Med. 2012;90:446–451.

18. Spagnolo J, Champagne F, Leduc N, Rivard M, Piat M, Laporta M, Melki W, Charfi F. Mental health knowledge, attitudes, and self-efficacy among primary care physicians working in the greater Tunis area of Tunisia. Int J Ment Health Syst. 2018;12:63. doi: 10.1186/s13033-018-0243-x.

19. Ben Thabet J, Mâalej M, Khemakhem H, Yaich S, Abbes W, Omri S, Zouari L, Zouari N, Dammak J, Charfi N, et al. The management of depressed patients by the Tunisian general practitioners: a critical trans-sectional study. Community Ment Health J. 2019;55:137–143. doi: 10.1007/s10597-018-0335-8.

CHAPTER 7

Depression and anxiety in primary care in Europe

DOI: 10.1201/9781003391531-7

7.1 DEPRESSION AND ANXIETY IN GREECE

Christos Lionis

Although a modern electronic record system has been developed in the Greek national health system, there is still a lack of data regarding the prevalence of the most frequent chronic diseases, including depression and anxiety. A representative sample of 4,894 individuals living in private households in Greece between 2009 and 2010 were assessed for common mental disorders in the past week using the revised Clinical Interview Schedule in a national survey.[1] Eleven percent of the male population and 14% of the female population were found to have clinically significant psychiatric morbidity. In another national representative sample of the adult population of Greece, 27% of the participants examined using a standardised protocol[2] reported symptoms relevant to anxiety and 16.7% to depression.[3] An anonymous online survey–based approach to estimate the prevalence of symptoms of psychological distress in the Greek population during the first COVID-19 lockdown had findings suggestive of high rates of depression, anxiety and post-traumatic stress disorder (PTSD) during that first lockdown.[4] Depression and anxiety symptoms in adolescents and young adults were also found frequently, associated with previous mental health history and co-existing attention/learning difficulties and substance use, rather than socioeconomic factors.[5]

These diagnoses are helpful. Frequently, Greek people interpret their symptoms as part of a physical disorder and there is a delay to seek care from primary care (PC) practitioners or specialists. Frequently patients will present to the doctor's office with somatic complaints and emotional feelings that they do not name as depression or anxiety, but as sadness or disappointment. This underlines the need to educate PC practitioners to work more on the medical interviewing, with a focus on feelings not traditionally included in the classification systems.

Although the current situation is rapidly changing in PC in Greece, with PC practitioners more involved in the diagnosis of mental health disorders, depression and anxiety, these disorders are still not routinely detected in primary care. A study of depression in a sample of elderly patients visiting a PC setting in rural Crete reported high rates of undetected depression of 61%.[6] This study found a prevalence of depression of 10.8% based on history or treatment of depression. However when an extensive neuropsychiatric/neuropsychological evaluation was used to define depression, the prevalence was 28.7% of the studied sample. Depression is also a frequent disorder in older people living in homes for elderly.

Practice guidelines for the management of depression and anxiety in PC based on an interdisciplinary consensus were approved six years ago in Greece. There is a stepped-care approach, and diagnostic algorithms are available at the Ministry of Health's website.[7] However, it is still unknown to what extent this guidance is implemented in daily practice. Integrated PC is still lacking in Greece, and policy recommendations were formulated in 2019 to guide primary health care reform in Greece, while attempting to inform efforts in other countries with similar conditions.[8]

A national action plan for Mental Health 2021–2030 has recently been approved, which includes actions for restructuring the Greek mental health services. The vertical axis No. 2 of this national plan stated "focusing on further development and integration of the community-based network of mental health services, while integrating mental health services into primary health care, using modern digital technologies".[9]

The residency programme in general practice in Greece includes specific training in psychiatry and mental health. Although there are efforts to increase training and the capacity of PC practitioners to detect depression and anxiety, there is substantial room for improvement. Training modules to respond to the current needs of PC practitioners in regard to depression and anxiety are needed. A retraining of all PC practitioners who serve the public sector is currently being planned by the Ministry of Health, and this will consist of online eLearning modules. The Medical Faculty at the University of Crete has developed a Primary Training Hub and begun developing a series of training courses, which it anticipated would be expanded upon. Activities that have been undertaken by the World Organization of Family Doctors (WONCA) Working Party on Mental Health are anticipated to enhance the existing capacity in PC in Greece.

REFERENCES

1. Skapinakis P, Bellos S, Koupidis S, Grammatikopoulos I, Theodorakis PN, Mavreas V. Prevalence and sociodemographic associations of common mental disorders in a nationally representative sample of the general population in Greece. BMC Psychiatry. 2013 Jun 4;13:163. doi: 10.1186/1471-244X-13-163
2. E.ME.NO. National Study of Morbidity and Risk Factors. 2023. Available from: https://www.beyondblue.org.au/ (accessed Mar 12, 2023).
3. Touloumi G, Karakatsani A, Karakosta A, et al. National survey of morbidity and risk factors (EMENO): protocol for a health examination survey representative of the adult Greek population. JMIR Res Protoc. 2019;8(2):e10997. doi: 10.2196/10997
4. Karaivazoglou K, Konstantopoulou G, Kalogeropoulou M, Iliou T, Vorvolakos T, Assimakopoulos K, et al. Psychological distress in the Greek general population during the first COVID-19 lockdown. BJ Psych Open. 2021;7:e59.
5. Basta M, Micheli K, Koutra K, Fountoulaki M, Dafermos V, Drakaki M, Faloutsos K, et al. Depression and anxiety symptoms in adolescents and young adults in Greece: prevalence and associated factors. J Affective Disord. 2022;8:100334. doi: 10.1016/j.jadr.2022.100334
6. Basta M, Micheli K, Simos P, Zaganas I, Panagiotakis S, Koutra K et al. Frequency and risk factors associated with depression in elderly visiting primary health care (PHC) settings: findings from the Cretan aging cohort. J Affect Disord. 2021; 4: 100109. doi: 10.1016/j.jadr.2021.100109

7. Ministry of Health. General Practice Guidelines for the Management of the Most Common Diseases in Primary Health Care. Mar 2017.

8. Lionis C, Symvoulakis EK, Markaki A, Petelos E, Papadakis S, Sifaki-Pistolla D, Papadakakis M, Souliotis K, Tziraki C. Integrated people-centred primary health care in Greece: unravelling Ariadne's thread. Prim Health Care Res Dev. Jul 25 2019;20:e113. doi: 10.1017/S1463423619000446

9. Hellenic Republic, Ministry of Health, National Mental Health Action Plan 2021–2030, Executive Summary, July 2022.

7.2 DEPRESSION AND ANXIETY IN LUXEMBOURG

Raquel Gómez Bravo

Luxembourg has a high overall proportion of prevalence of depressive symptoms of 11% in the population, which can be explained by the accessibility of the system, whereas the average in the European Union is lower. Before the pandemic, the prevalence of anxiety was 4.9%.[1] The COVID-19 pandemic and the confinement measures intensified both pathologies, with women and younger groups at a higher risk of anxiety and depression.[2,3]

The signs and symptoms described in the *Diagnostic and Statistical Manual of Mental Disorders, Fifth Edition* (DSM-5) and International Classification of Diseases (ICD-11) are the common presentations of anxiety and depression in the country.[4] A high percentage of patients complain of burnout in Luxembourg. Anxiety and depression as underlined health problems may not be diagnosed unless specifically asked about, and often patients tend to hide their symptoms. Depression is often accompanied by anxiety, and addictions or abuse are frequently linked to these pathologies as well. Unfortunately, under-detection is also common in elderly patients. It is crucial to address any symptoms as early as possible and make a differential diagnosis in order to offer the appropriate support due to the high impact on the individual, their families and their working or social environment.[5]

Depression and anxiety are not routinely screened for in primary care in Luxembourg. Case-finding is the norm, using validated questionnaires when there is a suspicion, but there is a lack of national protocols and standardised procedures. For depression, the most common used are the WHO-5 and the Patient Health Questionnaire for depression (PHQ-9). For anxiety, the Center for Epidemiologic Studies Depression Scale (CES-D Scale), Generalised Anxiety Disorder 7-item (GAD-7 scale), Loneliness Scale – Short Version (UCLA Scale) and Perceived Stress Scale 4-item version (PSS-4) may be used.

There is no coordinated strategy in place to routinely manage these pathologies in Luxembourg, although it is considered a priority. There is also self-testing available through the Ministry of Health website and awareness-raising campaigns in several languages, with useful information on how to proceed to seek help, listing the resources available in the country.[5] The Ministry of Health promotes health education campaigns, encouraging the public to self-test and to understand the nature of their symptoms (as self-management is an important part of tackling mental health issues). If the results are positive or people have any mental health concerns, the website offers all types of information about how to arrange an appointment with a general practitioner, referral to another specialist or a private consultation with a psychologist or psychotherapist. Moreover, the details of the different services, various support groups, helplines that offer psychological support and other resources, languages available and time schedules are detailed, as well as the offer to leave a message and be contacted in a maximum of three working days. Specific services for children and young people are also available, and special attention is given to emergencies and suicide prevention, guiding the population on how to get help for themselves or loved ones. There are 24-hour acute psychiatric services available in every hospital in the four regions of Luxembourg.

In June 2021, the Ministry of Health and Ligue d'Hygiène Mentale launched mental health first aid classes, with the aim of training 3% of the population by 2030. The classes teach, in different languages, how family, friends or co-workers can provide initial support for mental health problems.[6]

General practitioners and other healthcare professionals are regularly offered training courses and continuous medical education is also available on a volunteer basis, to detect and manage these health care problems and refer to the appropriate professionals to provide proper care and follow-up. However, there is a lack of formal coordination between the different health care services and care provided, with an added barrier to coordination being the absence of shared electronic health records between primary and secondary care.

There are three main types of treatment: Medical, psychological, and social, which are often combined. Medical treatment can be prescribed by doctors in primary care or psychiatry, and there is a tendency to provide pharmacological treatment directly, in that it is reimbursed by the National Health Fund (Caisse nationale de santé, CNS) at 80% of the cost. However, other treatment options are usually only applied in specialized centres, as most of the main hospitals have psychiatric units or clinics for outpatient and inpatient treatment, potentially combined with rehabilitation. Secondary care services may be offered on an individual basis or in small groups of patients whether they are hospitalized or receiving outpatient care.

Psychotherapy or psychological and psychosocial counselling can be used on its own or in combination with medication for worse cases, individually or in groups. It is supported by the CNS at hospitals and other institutions, although some services provided in private practice are not covered. However, from February 2023 on, psychotherapy will be partially reimbursed by the CNS (70% for adults and 100% for insureds who have not reached the age of 18 on the date the medical prescription is issued), which should reduce the waiting lists and increase the accessibility of care. Teleconsultation is available via e-Consult on e-Sante if patients cannot attend an appointment in person. The University of Luxembourg offers a mental well-being counselling service for students and employees in both physical and virtual formats.

Social and other interventions have a very important role. These include social activities, relaxation strategies, dietary changes if necessary, moderate regular exercise and medical leave when needed, promoting hope and empowerment that add to the therapeutic effect of the medical and psychological treatment. Social and other interventions have a very important role. These include social activities, relaxation strategies, dietary changes if necessary, moderate regular exercise and medical leave when needed, promoting hope and empowerment that add to the therapeutic effect of both the medical and psychological treatment. However, community-based care for patients with depression and anxiety could be improved. Central guidelines and national protocols that promote better coordination among health care professionals would improve the care of the patients, as would follow-up after hospital discharge, as there is no national surveillance available yet, nor a centralized prescriptions network and shared electronic health care records with unique patient identifiers.

Mental health is a priority of the government. As mentioned, the government has recently approved the reimbursement of psychotherapy by the CNS and the national mental health plan in July 2023. The plan outlines 26 objectives across six key areas: governance, information systems and research, human resources, health promotion, mental health care access, and vulnerable populations. It represents a significant step forward in mental health care, building on the previous psychiatry reform and the 2015-2019 national suicide prevention plan.

The national mental health plan aims to create a stigma-free mental health care system that's on par with physical health care, seamlessly integrated into the broader health system. The ministry envisions a system that fosters cooperation among all stakeholders, offering transparent coordination and accessibility to individuals of all ages and illness severity levels.

The plan's next steps involve its launch, the establishment of a national mental health committee, the implementation of its governance, and the formation of various working groups.

REFERENCES

1. Statistical Office of the European Union (Eurostat) Revision of the European Standard Population Report of Eurostat's Task Force – 2013 edition. Publications Office of the European Union, Luxembourg. 2013. Available from: https://ec.europa.eu/eurostat/web/products-manuals-and-guidelines/-/KS-RA-13-028 (As at 19.02.2019)
2. Ribeiro F, Schröder VE, Krüger R, Leist AK; CON-VINCE Consortium. The evolution and social determinants of mental health during the first wave of the COVID-19 outbreak in Luxembourg. Psychiatry Res. 2021;303:114090. doi: 10.1016/j.psychres. 2021. 114090
3. O'Connor KJ, Peroni C. One in three Luxembourg residents report their mental health declined during the COVID-19 crisis. Int J Community Wellbeing. 2021;4(3):345–51. doi: 10.1007/s42413-020-00093-4
4. World Health Organization. International classification of diseases (11th revision). 2022. https://icd.who.int/
5. Service Information et Prévention de la Ligue 2022. Screening for Depression. Available from: https://www.prevention-depression.lu/en/for-professionals/general-practitioners/screening-for-depression/
6. Portail d'information sur la santé mentale 2020–2023. Available from: https://www.prevention-psy.lu/formation/

7.3 DEPRESSION AND ANXIETY IN TÜRKIYE

Sabah Tuzun, Pemra Cöbek Ünalan and Saliha Serap Cifcili

According to the Turkey Mental Health Profile Study, 1998, 17.2% of the Turkish population suffered from a mental illness in the past 12 months, and the prevalence of major depressive disorder (MDD) was reported to be 4%.[1,2] The prevalence of MDD among the population over 15 years of age was 9%, as per the 2019 data from the Health Statistics of Türkiye.[3] In Turkey's Health Study, a 22.7% increase in the frequency of depression and a 22.9% increase in the frequency of anxiety disorder were reported in 2019 compared to 2002.[3,4] In a primary care study, 46.6% of the participants had at least one of the mental disorders evaluated with the PRIME-MD questionnaire.[5] In this study, the most common mental health disorders were found to be mood disorders (30.2%) and anxiety disorders (25.2%).[6] In another community-based study, the prevalence of at least one mood disorder in adult individuals was 37%, and the prevalence of an anxiety disorder was 29%.[7] The risk factors for mental disorders were being a housewife, being less educated, having low income or being unemployed.[5,7,8]

Family Health Centres (FHCs) and Healthy Life Centres (HLCs) are regarded as primary mental health care providers in Türkiye under the National Mental Health Action Plan. Accordingly, it is expected that family physicians would diagnose and intervene in common mental illnesses such as minor depression and anxiety and that HLCs would provide counselling and support services.[9] However, patients are free to present to all specialties in secondary and tertiary public health care facilities and in private practice (there is no gate-keeping role for family medicine). In fact, family physicians or nurses do not routinely screen their populations for depression and anxiety as part of usual medical care. However, numerous screening scales are available for depression and anxiety. One of the most frequently used scales for depression is the Beck Depression Scale.[10] The Ministry of Health does not recommend screening for depression or anxiety in primary care, although they do recommend screening older adults using the Yesavage Geriatric Depression Scale and the Hamilton Anxiety Scale.[11]

According to these Ministry of Health guidelines, patients who screen positive should be referred to a psychiatrist,[11] although primary care physicians might choose to provide treatment to their patients as well. Psychologists employed in HLCs also provide counselling for patients.

Additionally, the 'community-based mental health' model is used as part of the Health Transformation Programme.[12,13] This model aims to prevent patients with mental illnesses from becoming isolated from society and losing their functionality through hospitalisation, as well as meeting their needs and improving their capacity to live in society, with the ultimate goal of fully integrating these patients into the community as much as possible.[12,13] In this model Community Mental Health Centres (CMHCs) are the facilities where people with serious mental illnesses are treated and followed up on; patients and their families are informed; mental education, group or individual therapy is delivered; and if necessary, home care is provided through a mobile team. These centres collaborate with psychiatry clinics.[12,13] Teams working at CMHCs have a minimum of two nurses, one part-time psychologist and one social worker on staff; efforts are still being made to establish these teams.[9,12,13] Additionally, it was intended for family physicians to be in contact with the units providing psychiatry services for guidance and supervision.[9]

Türkiye's nationwide primary health care system and universal health insurance coverage are advantages in the delivery of mental health services. A national personal electronic health record system, e-nabız (e-pulse), enables primary care physicians to see all their patients' health records, if patients give informed consent, to enable improved coordination of care.[14] Türkiye also has a current National Mental Health Action Plan[9] which specifies several actions to be made to provide education to primary care health professionals. CMHCs, which are community-based treatment follow-up and rehabilitation services, add important value for mental health services. The Mental Health Act was prepared with the consensus of nine non-governmental organisations together with the Turkish Psychiatric Association and proposed in 2006.[15]

However, there are still several challenges regarding mental health services in primary care. Mental health is not among the prioritised services supported by incentives in primary care such as well-child visits and antenatal follow-ups. Although there is a well-established electronic health record system, there is no specific electronic patient recording system for primary mental health problems. Secondary mental health care services are not integrated with primary care.[16] There is no referral system; rather, family physicians advise their patients to make an appointment and consult with a specialist by themselves if needed.

In addition to the lack of vertical integration, the community-based mental health services, namely FHCs, HLCs, and CMHCs, are not integrated as well. CMHCs and HLCs work separately from FHCs, which causes fragmentation and weakens mental health services in primary care. Furthermore, the provision of HLCs is not yet completed. There are workforce issues, with a limited number of health professionals providing psychological counselling or social services in community-based mental health services. In addition, antidepressants prescribed by a primary care physician are reimbursed for only one month by the National Health Insurance System. After one month, the treatment is reimbursed only if a report is provided by a psychiatrist.

Considering these challenges, several future acts could improve primary care mental health services. Although the latest version of the Mental Health Act was submitted to the Turkish Grand National Assembly as a law proposal in 2018, it has yet to be enacted.[17] Finalising this law will be a valuable contribution to primary mental health services in Türkiye. The resources of HLCS and CMHS should be augmented by integrating their operation with FHCs. In addition, a well-constructed referral system should be described and supported with electronic records to establish vertical integration of mental health services. Primary mental health care services could be supported with incentives, and barriers to treatment, such as limitations on reimbursements, could be cancelled.

REFERENCES

1. Coskun B. Psychiatry in Turkey. Int Psychiatry. 2004;1(3):13–15.
2. Kılıc C, Rezaki M, Ustun TB, Gater RA. Pathways to psychiatric care in Ankara. Soc Psychiatry Psychiatr Epidemiol. 1994;29:131–36.
3. Bora Basara B, Soytutan Caglar İ, Aygun A, Ozdemir TA, Kulali B. Health Statistics Yearbook 2020:35–53 [Internet]. General Directorate of Health Information Systems, Ministry of Health of Türkiye, Ankara 2022. Available from: https://sbsgm.saglik.gov.tr/Eklenti/43400/0/siy2020-eng-26052022pdf.pdf. (accessed 29 January 2023).
4. Turkish Statistical Institute. Turkey's Health Research 2019. [cited Nov 29, 2023]. https://data.tuik.gov.tr/Kategori/GetKategori?p=Saglik-ve-Sosyal-Koruma-101.
5. Dönmez L, Dedeoğlu N, Özcan E. Psychological disorders among primary health care patients. Turk Psikiyatri Derg. 2000;11(3):198–203. Turkish.
6. Keskin A, Unluoglu I, Bilge U, Yenilmez C. The prevalence of psychiatric disorders distribution of subjects gender and its relationship with psychiatric help-seeking. Noro Psikiyatr Ars. 2013;50:344–51.
7. Ogel K, Ozmen E, Boratav C. Depression in primary health care. Turk Psikiyatri Derg. 2000;11(1):3–16. Turkish.
8. Topuzoglu A, Binbay T, Ulas H, Elbi H, Aksu Tanık F, Zagli N, et al. The epidemiology of major depressive disorder and subthreshold depression in Izmir, Turkey: prevalence, socioeconomic differences, impairment, and help-seeking. J Affect Disord. 2015;181:78–86.
9. Ministry of Health, Republic of Turkey. National Mental Health Action Plan 2020–2023. [cited Nov 29, 2023]. Turkish.
10. Kılınç S, Torun F. Depression rating scales used in clinical practice in Turkey. Dirim. 2011;86(1):39–47. Turkish.
11. Ministry of Health. Republic of Turkey. General Directorate of Public Health. Periodic Health Examinations and Screening Tests Recommended in Family Medicine Practice Ankara, 2015. Report No: 991. [cited Nov 29, 2023]. Turkish.
12. Bilge A, Mermer G, Çam MO, Çetinkaya A, Erdoğan E, Üçkuyu N. Profile of community mental health centers in Turkey between 2013–2015 years. KOU Sag Bil Derg. 2016;2(2):1–5. Turkish.
13. Tirgil A, Hızıroğlu A. Mental health determinants in Turkey: investigating an extensive list of variables. J Humanity Soc. 2021;11(2):47–69.
14. Turkish National Personal Health Record System: e-pulse. [cited Jan 29, 2023]. Available from: https://wsa-global.org/winner/turkish-national-personal-health-record-system-e-pulse/.

15. Caglar E, Kaser M. Mental health law in Turkey: legislation pending. Int Psychiatry. 2014;11(1):12–14.

16. Cicekoglu P, Duran S. Community Based Preventive Mental Health Care Services in Turkey and in the World. In: Toplum Ruh Sağlığı Hemşireliği Ünsal Barlas G, editors 1. Edition, Ankara; Türkiye Klinikleri 2018. p. 8–14. Turkish.

17. Oncu F. Turkey's exam with mental health act. Toplum ve Hekim. 2020;35(4):316–20. Turkish.

7.4 DEPRESSION AND ANXIETY IN THE UNITED KINGDOM

Amanda Howe

The prevalence of depression and anxiety in the United Kingdom (UK) is currently cited in the most recent governmental survey as one in six (17%) reporting a common mental health problem, about half of which were specified as depression or anxiety.[1] Another study showed that the average lifetime prevalence of depression was 14.6% for adults, with an average 12-month prevalence estimate of 5.5%.[2] Many studies show that mental health problems are more common in women in all age groups and that those who are economically or socially disadvantaged are also more at risk of mental health problems and their adverse consequences. The COVID-19 pandemic was shown to increase mental health symptoms, but the overall prevalence of actual mental health disorders has not yet been shown to be greatly increased.

How depression and anxiety manifest in the UK somewhat depends on the context of the person involved, as does the language used to describe these conditions. Standardised clinical screening tools such as the commonly used Patient Health Questionnaire (PHQ-9)[3] and Generalized Anxiety Disorder assessment (GAD-7)[4] use very different words and tones from, for example, a mental health charity website which is trying to give a voice to lay people.[5] Similarly, the prevalence of psychological symptoms is much higher than condition-specific diagnoses – for example, material from the Royal College of General Practitioners (RCGP) estimates significant psychological issues are relevant in up to 40% of general practitioner (GP) consultations, but not all of these will reach diagnostic criteria.

However, both making an accurate assessment of psychological aspects and making specific diagnoses such as depression and anxiety disorders are routine parts of primary care in the UK.[6] The first step in the process is either patients themselves cite a psychological issue as their cause for consultation or their friends and family encourage them to present this if they perceive a problem. Staff in primary care are trained to routinely enquire about how people are feeling and also to detect psychological problems. Once these cues are raised, questions similar to those in the two common screening tools cited earlier will be used to make a firmer diagnosis, though this is more commonly done verbally than through the completion of a manual questionnaire.

The management of significant psychological problems may be 'expectant waiting and self-help advice' in the first instance, as the therapeutic impact of disclosure and empathic response can in itself start to increase insight and enable improvement. Patients would normally be offered a follow-up appointment with a suitable member of staff, and those with persistent problems will usually be offered one of three interventions – talking therapies, medications or referral to specialist mental health services if appropriate. The first of these is the most common next step in the UK, and indeed patients can refer themselves online to the National Health Service (NHS) services without a GP referral if they already understand what they might need.[7] Medication is a common next step if symptoms are severe or prolonged, and psychiatric referrals made for those who have very severe symptoms or deterioration.

During the last 40 years in the UK, increasing attention has been paid to both 'health literacy'[8] (the personal characteristics and social resources needed for individuals and communities to access, understand, appraise and use information and services to make positive decisions about health) and emotional literacy (the ability to recognise, understand, handle and express emotions). In principle, this should help our population recognise psychological problems and seek help promptly if needed. However, societal factors can influence this – mental health remains relatively stigmatised in many cultures; our diverse population with its many backgrounds may have different perceptions of what constitutes mental health and how to discuss it; and concern about the reactions of others to any admission of psychological problems can also be a barrier. Sadly, socioeconomic divisions are currently widening in our country, and this is also impacting on mental health from childhood onwards.

In primary care, mental health is core business, and all staff now have some training to alert them to these problems. National bodies such as the RCGP also provide clear leadership as to the importance of mental health in core primary care, with an approach that goes wider than just depression and anxiety into multiple other diagnoses and the need for integrated and effective services.[9] However, the aim to engage sensitively with all and to diagnose psychological issues may be jeopardised by workload and limitations on time and energy.

In addition, government reports show that while funding and workforce for mental health services have increased, as have the number of people being treated, there will still be 'sizeable treatment gaps' by 2023–2024 if further action is not taken.[10] Some key facts show that 4.5 million people were in contact with NHS-funded mental health services during 2021–2022, and £12 billion was spent on mental health services in 2021–2022, equivalent to around 9% of the NHS budget.[11] There is also increased need – there was a 44% increase in referrals to NHS mental health services between 2016–2017 and 2021–2022, from 4.4 million in 2016–2017 to 6.4 million in 2021–2022. Need also outstrips service capacity, with 1.2 million estimated people on the waiting list for community-based NHS mental health services at the end of June 2022 and with some areas not yet recognised – for example, the proportion of referrals to talking therapy services is currently excluded from the calculation of waiting time standards.

So to summarise – the UK NHS, and primary care within it, offer care for depression and anxiety that should be easy to access, of high quality and free at the point of use, with a reduction in cultural barriers that is also helpful. But excellent diagnosis and management can be impacted by wider societal challenges, increasing prevalence and the current stress in the NHS following years of reorganisations and increasing workload. We hope for better times.

REFERENCES

1. Baker C, Kirk-Wade E. Mental Health Statistics: prevalence, services and funding In England. Commons Library Research Briefing. March 2023. Available from: https://commonslibrary.parliament.uk/research-briefings/sn06988/ (accessed May 12, 2023).
2. National Institute for Health and Care Excellence. Depression Guideline. 2023. Available from: https://cks.nice.org.uk/topics/depression/background-information/prevalence/ (accessed May 12, 2023).
3. Patient Health Questionnaire PHQ-9. Available from: PHQ-9 Depression Test Questionnaire | Patient (accessed May 12, 2023).
4. Generalised Anxiety Disorder Assessment GAD-7. Available from: GAD7 Anxiety Test Questionnaire | Patient (accessed May 12, 2023).
5. MIND U.K. National Charity. Common signs and Symptoms of Depression. Available from: https://www.mind.org.uk/information-support/types-of-mental-health-problems/depression/symptoms/#CommonSignsAndSymptomsOfDepression (accessed May 12, 2023).
6. NHS Homepage on Mental Health. Available from: https://www.nhs.uk/mental-health/ (accessed May 12, 2023).
7. NHS Guidance on Talking Therapies. Available from: https://www.hee.nhs.uk/our-work/mental-health/improving-access-psychological-therapies (accessed May 12, 2023).
8. NHS. Definition of Health Literacy. Available from: https://www.england.nhs.uk/personalisedcare/health-literacy (accessed May 12, 2023).
9. Royal College of General Practitioners, U.K. Mental Health Clinical Toolkit. Available at: Mental health toolkit: Introduction (rcgp.org.uk) (accessed May 12, 2023).
10. Mehase E. Government must get a grip on mental health crisis. BMJ. 2023;380:324. doi: 10.1136/bmj.p324
11. National Audit Office, Progress in Improving Mental Health Services in England. 2023. Available from: https://www.nao.org.uk/wp-content/uploads/2023/02/Progress-in-improving-mental-health-services-CS.pdf (accessed May 12, 2023).

CHAPTER 8

Depression and anxiety in primary care in Ibero-Americana

DOI: 10.1201/9781003391531-8

8.1 DEPRESSION AND ANXIETY IN ARGENTINA

Lidia Caballero, Matías Tonnelier and Silvia Reina

In recent studies carried out in the Argentinean population, the lifetime prevalence of any mental disorder in the general population over 18 years of age was 29% and the projected life risk up to the age of 75 was 37%.[1] The disorders with the highest life prevalence were major depressive disorder (8.7%), alcohol abuse disorder (8.1%) and specific phobia (6.8%). Anxiety disorders were the most prevalent group (16.4%), followed by mood disorders (12.3%), substance disorders (10.4%) and impulse control disorders (2.5%). The prevalence in the last 12 months of any mental disorder was 14.8%, a quarter of which were classified as severe. A reported 11.6% received treatment in the previous 12 months, and only 30.2% of those who suffered from a severe disorder received treatment for it.[2,3]

Depression is underdiagnosed in Argentina – it is not recognised or well-treated because of psychic masking hiding behind anxiety; somatic masking with the appearance of pain or its increase; or comorbidity with other conditions, whether psychiatric, neurological or clinical.[4] Anxiety may manifest as generalised anxiety disorder, panic disorder or specific phobias and including social phobia.[2]

Tools to diagnose depression and anxiety are not routinely used in daily practice, and detection requires primary health professionals to be attentive to symptoms of them. A multistage probabilistic survey of the Composite International Diagnostic Interview (CIDI) designed by the World Health Organization has been used in research settings. The CIDI is a fully structured diagnostic interview used in the World Mental Health Survey Initiative, which includes Spanish-speaking countries in Latin America.[5] The disorders were evaluated using the diagnostic criteria of the *Diagnostic and Statistical Manual of Mental Disorders, Fourth Edition* (DSM-IV).[2]

Argentina adheres to the international frameworks of Integral Management for Disaster Risk Reduction (GIRRD), enacting Law No. 27,287, which created the National System for Integral Risk Management and Civil Protection (SINAGIR). The Inter-Agency Standing Committee (IASC) proposes a pyramid of interventions for mental health and psychosocial support teams that illustrates different levels of support. For the purposes of the COVID-19 emergency context, the pyramid has been adapted from the 2007 pyramid.[6]

Management of depression includes pharmacological treatments that may or may not be accompanied by non-pharmacological treatments. Behavioural and cognitive behavioural therapy are the predominant non-pharmacological treatments, either alone or in combination with pharmacological management.[7] There are currently two behavioural activation formats or models for therapy: the Behavioural Activation model (BA) and the Brief Activation

Treatment for Depression model (BATD).[8] The differences between the two are relatively minor: They are based on different learning principles; BATD is more structured than BA; BA incorporates elements of functional analysis and tools for dealing with rumination, whereas BATD focuses exclusively on behavioural activation.[9]

For the treatment of anxiety, selective serotonin uptake inhibitors are mainly used, as well as high-potency benzodiazepines, such as clonazepam, used mainly in the initial period of treatment to attenuate autonomic activation symptoms and overcome anticipatory anxiety in the face of feared situations.[10]

The majority of patients with depression are not prescribed any medication, and only 31% receive antidepressants.[4] Within pharmacological treatments, the useful daily doses for social anxiety disorder generally range from 20–40 mg of fluoxetine or paroxetine, 50–100 mg of sertraline, 100–200 mg of fluvoxamine or 10–20 mg of escitalopram.[10]

The IASC guidelines propose a series of levels of interventions (stepped care) for the different health agents for 'Mental Health and Psychosocial Support in Humanitarian Emergencies and Disasters'. These include:

1. *Basic services and security*:
   - Risk communication
   - Promotion of protection measures, security, information and response to basic needs and psychosocial aspects

2. *Community and family support*:
   - Basic mental health care by primary care personnel
   - *Adapted psychological first aid*: By health care professionals in person or remotely

3. *Non-specialised (person-to-person) focused support*:
   - *Adapted psychological first aid*: By community agents
   - Mutual support and other community psychosocial strategies
   - Information with recommendations for vulnerable groups

4. *Specialised services*:
   - Guidance, accompaniment, mental health counselling and psychosocial support in person or by teleconsultation
   - On-site emergency care (when necessary)
   - Continuity of care and follow-up of pre-existing treatments, including the pharmacological plan through the incorporation of digital prescriptions[6]

The guidelines for the implementation of the Mental Health Law N26.657, with a plan that covers the period 2021–2025, arises in the context of a scenario marked by the health emergency caused by the COVID-19 pandemic. Thus, Argentina has now included in its public health agenda a series of steps to strengthen the diagnosis, follow-up and treatment of the mental health of its population.[11] The National Mental Health Plan 2021/2025, in particular its Problem No. 5, proposes continuous in-service training of human resources in health/mental health for the different sectors involved.[11]

The current crisis situation due to COVID 19 is an invaluable opportunity for the urgent implementation of care strategies, which should contemplate at least the following three basic dimensions: Training, promotion and organisational strategies.[5]

REFERENCES

1. World Health Organization. *Depression and other common mental disorders: global health estimates.* Geneva; 2017. License: CC BY-NC-SA 3.0 IGO.
2. Stagnaro JC, Cía A, Vázquez N, Vommaro H, Nemirovsky M, Serfaty E, Sustas SE, Medina Mora ME, Benjet C, Aguilar-Gaxiola S, Kessler R. Estudio epidemiológico de salud mental en población general de la República Argentina. VERTEX Rev Arg de Psiquiat. 2018;29:275–99.
3. Cía AH, Stagnaro JC, Aguilar Gaxiola S. et al Lifetime prevalence and age-of-onset of mental disorders in adults from the Argentinean study of mental health epidemiology. Soc Psychiatry Psychiatr Epidemiol. 2018;53:341–50.
4. Rojtenberg S. Depresiones en atención primaria. Ciudad Autónoma de Buenos Aires: Laboratorio Gador; 2019.
5. Pan American Health Organization. Considerations and Recommendations for Protecting the Healthcare Teams' Mental Health. 2021. This work is available under the CC BY-NC-SA 3.0 IGO license.
6. Guía del IASC sobre Salud Mental y Apoyo Psicosocial en Emergencias Humanitarias y Catástrofes https://www.acnur.org/media/guia-del-iasc-sobre-salud-mental-y-apoyo-psicosocialen-emergencias-humanitarias-y-catastrofes Adaptación de la pirámide de la Guía del IASC sobre Salud Mental y Apoyo Psicosocial en Emergencias Humanitarias y Catástrofes del 2007 en Junio 2020. [cited February 25, 2023].
7. Cía AH. Tratamiento de la ansiedad en la Clínica y en la Atención Primaria: ansiedad/Alfredo H. Cía. Ciudad Autónoma de Buenos Aires: Laboratorio Gador; 2019.
8. Lejuez CW, Hopko DR, Hopko SD. A brief behavioral activation treatment for depression. Treatment manual. Behav Modif. 2001;25(2):255–286.
9. Maero F. Activación conductual: Un tratamiento simple y eficaz para la depresión. 2012. PSYCIENCIA. [cited February 15, 2023]. Available from: https://www.psyciencia.com/activacion-conductual-un-tratamiento-simple-y-eficaz-para-la-depresion-2/
10. Cía AH. Trastorno de Ansiedad Social-Manual Diagnóstico, Terapéutico y de Autoayuda, Editorial Polemos, Buenos Aires. 2005.
11. Argentina. Se presentó el Plan Nacional de Salud Mental 2021/2025. [cited February 24, 2023]. Available from: https://www.argentina.gob.ar/noticias/se-presento-el-plan-nacional-de-salud-mental-20212025

8.2 DEPRESSION AND ANXIETY IN BRAZIL

Adelson Guaraci Jantsch

Like many countries that transitioned their morbimortality patterns, Brazil has today a high prevalence of all chronic conditions among its adult population. However, the epidemiological transition in Brazil was not as complete as seen in high-income countries, since the country still struggles with high rates of death due to communicable diseases, car crashes and violent acts.[1,2] At the same time, with improvements in living standards and the increasing life expectancy (from 49.5 years in 1950 to 76.5 years in 2022), all chronic conditions followed the same patterns as countries that underwent a complete epidemiological transition.[3] Mental health conditions, including depression and anxiety, became more common in Brazilian society. Alcohol abuse and tobacco dependency remain highly prevalent, despite the lower prevalence in younger generations, probably due to public campaigns aiming to reduce access to alcohol and tobacco among teenagers.[4]

Global health estimates put Brazil as the world leader in the prevalence of anxiety disorders and second place in depression, just behind the United States.[5] One explanation is the increase in number of years lived with disability, especially in young adults.[6] National surveys have shown that the prevalence of adults with depression – both self-reported or evaluated with the Patient Health Questionnaire-9 (PHQ-9) – has increased from 7.5% in 2013 to 10% in 2019, with an even higher prevalence among those who are sedentary, tobacco smokers, heavy drinkers and young unemployed adults.[7] Seeking health care for depression also increased during this period from 46% to 53% among those self-reporting as having depression, with private clinics being the main source of health care.[8]

The words depression and anxiety are not restricted to the medical vocabulary in Brazil. They are already part of the vernacular Portuguese, along with other terms commonly used by patients to describe symptoms of anxiety and depression, such as *"estar com nervos"* (being nervous), *"tristeza"* (sadness), *"estar com os nervos à flor da pele"* (be on edge), *"me sinto muito agitado/agitada"* (I am feeling very agitated or hectic) and *"estou com muita ansiedade"* (I am having a lot of anxiety). Of course, patients will use their own words to describe their own illness experience, with many using expressions such as "Doctor, I am depressed" or "I am feeling very anxious". Many will tell a different story, such as "Doctor, I want to be happy again", said a young nanny starting to realise that her beloved employers were making her work overtime taking care of their children without paying for it. Or "I miss the smell of the rain in my little farm in Ceará", said an old woman after three months of living in a favela in Rio de Janeiro against her will, but trying to please her daughter who gratefully wanted to give her mother the rest she deserved after a whole life dedicated to the family.

In order to improve detection and management skills of health profession-als in primary care, the Brazilian Ministry of Health has led several initia-tives to increase the scope of practice of doctors and nurses, including the publication of guidelines, guiding manuals and online courses on mental health problems.[9] This capacity-building approach has focused on creating a more holistic approach to illness, avoiding overprescription of psychotropics, unnecessary referrals to secondary care and hospital admissions. Standard screening tools are used to diagnose depression and anxiety and are avail-able by most of the digital platforms doctors often use on a daily basis. These screening and diagnostic tools are taught in medical schools and in continu-ous medical education courses. Despite these efforts, trends in the sales of antidepressants in Brazil have increased from 2014 to 2020.[10] This information raises concerns regarding the possibility that many patients using antidepres-sants and anxiolytics are not taking them to treat depression or anxiety, but may be over-diagnosed and/or over-treated for something else.

The Brazilian Psychiatric Reform was initiated in the 1980s and formally established in 2001 with the publication of the Psychiatric Reform Law.[11] It was a comprehensive reform that changed not only the way patients with schizophrenia and psychosis were treated so far (mostly in long stays in psy-chiatric hospitals, before the reform, away from their families and communi-ties). With the community becoming the main setting for treating all mental health conditions, primary care became responsible for being the first contact and the main resource in the community to take care of patients with all sorts of mental health issues.[12]

The Brazilian Family Health Strategy – the first national initiative for pri-mary health care – was launched in 1994.[13] It established a model of care, a governance structure and financial incentives for municipalities to implement Family Health Teams – a team of health workers (one physician, one nurse, one nurse technician and four to six community health agents) taking care of 4,000 people living in a catchment area. Today, this strategy is responsible for providing primary care to 66% of the population.[14,15] Coordination of care starts in primary care for all health issues, not only mental health. One patient with depression and/or anxiety can be diagnosed and managed a in a primary care clinic by his or her Family Health Team, but quite often many patients are referred to psychiatrists to be managed, mostly those with schizophrenia, psychotic symptoms or severe cases.

The reform was also followed by two national initiatives that helped opera-tionalise the reform and make it reach its goals. The first was the expansion of the Psychosocial Support Center (*Centros de Apoio Psicosocial* – CAPS) to provide improved access to mental health care in the community, allowing routine visits and follow-up of patients by health care teams and combining the expertise of psychologists, psychiatrists, nurses, occupational therapists, music therapists and other professionals. The second was the creation of the Nucleus of Support for the Family Health Strategy (Núcleo de Apoio à Saúde da Família – NASF)[16] that allowed municipalities to create health care teams with other health professionals than those already available in Family Health Teams – general doctors and nurses. This initiative brought to primary care the expertise of nutritionists, physiotherapists, occupational therapists and psychologists. The work of health professionals from NASF is meant primarily to support Family Health Teams manage their patients through shared consultations, shared decision-making and case discussions.[17] They also have their own patients and one agenda jointly created with the Family Health Teams. Ultimately, this initiative has improved access to health care for patients with depression and anxiety. By 2023, there were 2,836 CAPS in all states of the country, totalling an annual funding of more than 1.27 billion Brazilian reais (250 million US dollars).

For the last 20 years, residency training in family medicine has been incentivised and expended by the Brazilian government.[18] Three waves of national policies aiming to promote the provision, fixation and training of doctors to work in primary care in rural and remote areas have helped to improve access to health care and, at the same time, improve primary care capacity to deal with depression, anxiety and other mental health issues.[19-21]

After two years of residency training in family medicine, Brazilian family physicians are more capable of detecting schizophrenia, psychosis, alcohol dependency, drug addictions, depression and anxiety, compared to doctors without residency training.[22] They also request fewer referrals to psychiatrists for these patients, managing them closely to the place where they live.[23] However, only a small portion of all 45,000 Family Health Teams in the country has a trained family physician. The majority of these teams have a generalist (a doctor with six years of medical school), who frequently spends the first years of his or her career working in primary care, before moving to another medical specialty.[24] Hopefully, with all efforts combined and in the next 10 years, this scenario will change and the majority of the Brazilian population will have one trained family physician – or at least one doctor with some training in family medicine – as their medical provider. This will represent an improvement in the quality of care provided to the communities and to all patients with mental health conditions.

REFERENCES

1. Peixoto SV. The triple burden of health problems and the challenges for the unified health system. Cien Saude Colet. 2020;25(8):2913. doi: 10.1590/1413-81232020258.14672020
2. Duarte EC, Barreto SM. Transição demográfica e epidemiológica: a Epidemiologia e Serviços de Saúde revisita e atualiza o tema. Epidemiol e Serviços Saúde. 2012;21(4): 529–32.

3. Marinho F, de Azeredo Passos VM, Carvalho Malta D, et al. Burden of disease in Brazil, 1990–2016: a systematic subnational analysis for the global burden of disease study 2016. Lancet. 2018;392. doi: 10.1016/S0140-6736(18)31221-2

4. Sanchez ZM, Oliveira Prado MC, Sanudo A, Carlini EA, Nappo SA, Martins SS. Trends in alcohol and tobacco use among Brazilian students: 1989 to 2010. Rev Saude Publica. 2015;49. doi: 10.1590/S0034-8910.2015049005860

5. World health Organization. Depression and other common mental disorders: global health estimates. Geneva; 2017. https://apps.who.int/iris/bitstream/handle/10665/254610/WHO-MSD-MER-2017.2-eng.pdf?sequence=1&isAllowed=y.

6. Bonadiman CSC, Malta DC, De Azeredo Passos VM, Naghavi M, Melo APS. Depressive disorders in Brazil: results from the global burden of disease study 2017. Popul Health Metr. 2020;18(Suppl 1):1–13. doi: 10.1186/s12963-020-00204-5

7. de Souza Lopes C, Gomes NL, Junger WL, Menezes PR. Trend in the prevalence of depressive symptoms in Brazil: results from the Brazilian national health survey 2013 and 2019. Cad Saude Publica. 2022;38:1–17. doi: 10.1590/0102-311X00123421

8. De Albuquerque Brito VC, Bello-Corassa R, Stopa S, Vasconcelossardinha L, Dahl C, Viana M. Prevalence of self-reported depression in Brazil: national health survey 2019 and 2013. Epidemiol e Serv Saude. 2022;31(Special issue 1):1–12. doi: 10.1590/SS2237-9622202200006.especial

9. Departamento de Atenção Básica; Brasil; Ministério da Saúde; Secretaria de Atenção à Saúde. *Cadernos de Atenção Básica, No 34 (Saúde Mental).* Vol 20. Brasília; 2013. doi: 10.29327/555654.1-5

10. Hoefler R, Tiguman GMB, Galvão TF, Ribeiro-Vaz I, Silva MT. Trends in sales of antidepressants in Brazil from 2014 to 2020: a time trend analysis with joinpoint regression. J Affect Disord. 2023;323:213–18. doi: 10.1016/J.JAD.2022.11.069

11. Brasil. Presidência da República. Casa Civil. Subchefia para Assuntos Jurídicos. *LEI No 10.216, DE 6 DE ABRIL DE 2001.* Brasília; 2001. http://www.planalto.gov.br/ccivil_03/leis/leis_2001/l10216.htm.

12. Hirdes A. A reforma psiquiátrica no Brasil: uma (re)visão. Cien Saude Colet. 2009;14(1):297–305.

13. Macinko J, Harris MJ. Brazil's family health strategy — delivering community-based primary care in a universal health system. N Engl J Med. 2015;372(23):2177–2181. doi: 10.1056/NEJMp1501140

14. Neves RG, Flores TR, Manjourany SSD, Nunes BP, Tomasi E. Time trend of family health strategy coverage in Brazil, its regions and federative units, 2006–2016. Epidemiol Serv Saude. 2016;27(34):1–8. doi: 10.5123/S1679-49742018000300008

15. Macinko J, de Fátima Marinho de Souza M, Guanais FC, da Silva Simões CC. Going to scale with community-based primary care: an analysis of the family health program and infant mortality in Brazil, 1999–2004. Soc Sci Med. 2007;65(10). doi: 10.1016/j.socscimed.2007.06.028

16. Brasil. Ministério da Saúde. *PORTARIA No 154, DE 24 DE JANEIRO DE 2008. Cria Os Núcleos de Apoio à Saúde Da Família - NASF.* 2008.

17. Gonçalves DA, Ballester D, Chiaverini DH, et al. *Guia Prático de Matriciamento Em Saúde Mental.* Vol 16. Brasília: Ministério da Saúde; 2011. doi: 10.54620/cadesp.v16i3.829

18. Sarti TD, Fontenelle LF, Gusso GDF. Panorama da expansão dos programas de Residência Médica em Medicina de Família e Comunidade no Brasil: desafios para sua consolidação. Rev Bras Med Família e Comunidade. 2018;13(40):1–5. doi: 10.5712/rbmfc13(40)1744

19. Brasil. *Portaria Interministerial N° 2.087, de 1° de Setembro de 2011. Institui o Programa de Valorização Do Profissional Da Atenção Básica. Diário Oficial Da União 2011; 2 Set.* 2011.

20. Brasil. *Lei 12.871 de 22 de Outubro de 2013. Institui o Programa Mais Médicos, Altera as Leis No 8.745, de 9 de Dezembro de 1993, e No 6.932, de 7 de Julho de 1981, e Dá Outras Providências.* Presidência da República; Casa Civil; Subchefia para Assuntos Jurídicos. 2013. http://www.planalto.gov.br/ccivil_03/_ato2011-2014/2013/lei/l12871.htm.

21. Brasil. *Medida Provisória N° 890, de 2019 (Programa Médicos Pelo Brasil).* Brasília: Comissão Mista da Medida Provisória n° 890, de 2019. 2019. https://www.congressonacional.leg.br/materias/medidas-provisorias/-/mpv/137836.

22. Jantsch AG, Burström B, Nilsson G, Leon APD. Detection and follow-up of chronic health conditions in Rio de Janeiro – the impact of residency training in family medicine. BMC Fam Pract. 2021;22(223):1–11. doi: 10.1186/s12875-021-01542-5

23. Jantsch AG, Burström B, Nilsson GH, Leon APD. Residency training in family medicine and its impact on coordination and continuity of care: an analysis of referrals to secondary care in Rio de Janeiro. BMJ Open. 2022;12:1–9. doi: 10.1136/bmjopen-2021-051515

24. Mário S. *Demografia Médica No Brasil 2020.* São Paulo: FMUSP & CFM; 2020.

8.3 DEPRESSION AND ANXIETY IN ECUADOR

Miriann Mora Verdugo, Diana López and Yolanda Dávila

The distribution of people in Ecuador is organised into 24 provinces, distributed into four large regions: Galapagos Islands, Highlands, Amazonia and Coast. According to self-identification, there is a large cultural diversity. The most representative nationality is Kichwa.[1]

In 2017, the World Health Organization (WHO) reported that Ecuador ranked eleventh in the world with cases of depression with a prevalence of 4.6% and tenth for anxiety with a prevalence of 5.6%.[2] Between 1990 and 2019, the prevalence of depression was 2.8% in men and 4.1% in women and anxiety was 4.1% in men and 6.8% in women.[3] In a study of a university population with a mean age of 18.3 years, 53.7% were women and 95.1% were mestizos (people of mixed European and indigenous ancestry). The prevalence of major depression was 6.2% and generalised anxiety was 2.2%.[4]

Dávila and collaborators, in a study of the Nabón canton, in the Ecuadorian Andes, which has a 30% indigenous population, found that the prevalence of depression in the total population was 4.5%. Of these, 67% were female, 30% were indigenous and 8% belonged to dysfunctional families. Also, 33% of people with major depression were aged 20–45 years. The prevalence of generalised anxiety was 8% among women, of whom 51% were between 20 and 42 years old, and 39% corresponded to the indigenous ethnic group. In another study of an older population with a median age of 70 years, the overall prevalence of depression was 35.4%. Of these, mild depression was 23.7%, moderate 8.7%, severe 3% and moderate/severe was 11.7%.[5]

Depression and anxiety constitute a public health problem. Three universities in the city of Cuenca found that 61% of their students, average age of 21 years, had this disorder.[6] Furthermore, many people with depression and anxiety present in medical consultations with physical symptoms such as pain, inability to sleep, eating behaviour problems and crying easily. In Ecuador, the Ministry of Public Health implemented the Comprehensive Care Model in Family and Community Health, strengthening primary health care, especially at the first level of care, which is responsible for detecting and treating 85% of the more frequent pathologies. The pillar for the application of the model is the family doctor. Mental health is also prioritised, integrating psychologists into health teams that cover a population of more than 10,000 people, but leaving a void for this service in communities with smaller populations. In these places, a problem arises when a mental disorder is detected, as they must be referred due to a lack of medication or psychologists, but patients must wait one or two months to be seen. Only if the mental illness is serious or the patient's life is at risk may they be referred with a priority or emergency shift to a specialised centre. Another problem is the belief that people have that if you go to the psychologist, it is because you are crazy, so they do not attend the consultation.

The Ministry of Public Health of Ecuador issued a Clinical Practice Guide, "Diagnosis and Treatment of Depressive Episode and Recurrent Depressive Disorder in Adults", in 2017 that must be applied at all levels of health.[7] It indicates that those with unexplained physical symptoms, chronic pain, fatigue, insomnia, anxiety and substance use are at greater risk of depression and gives general recommendations for the suspicion and screening of depression in adults.

For the diagnosis of depression, the criteria of the International Classification of Diseases (ICD-10) are used. Once the problem is identified, the severity criteria of a depressive episode are applied, and together with the diagnosis or suspicion of depression, physical and mental comorbidities must be ruled out, which may be associated with substances and medications. A detailed anamnesis, physical and psychological examination, and laboratory tests are required in patients with a suspicion or diagnosis of depression. These tests include basal glycemia, thyroxine (T_4), thyroid-stimulating hormone (TSH) and others based on medical criteria. "Scales can be used to provide complementary information in the evaluation, but they cannot replace the clinical interview". They recommend the validated Spanish version of the Hamilton Rating Scale for Depression (HRSD or HAM-D), as well as the validated Spanish version of the Montgomery-Asberg Depression Rating Scale (MADRS) and the Beck Depression Inventory (BDI-13 and 21-item versions). There is no guide for the diagnosis or management of anxiety. This diagnosis is made based on signs and symptoms.

As the first level of care, the gateway to the system and the first point of contact with the population, family and community health units are the location where the greatest number of screenings and detections of people with mental health problems are performed, particularly by family doctors. During the consultation, risk factors are determined for people with chronic diseases; a history of depressive episodes; a family history of depression; and problems such as unemployment, spousal separation, stressful life events, violence, alcohol consumption, fibromyalgia, chronic fatigue, etc.

Ideally once the diagnosis is established, interdisciplinary treatment begins, which consists of a proportion of interventions based on the patient's state and evolution, such as referring the patient to psychological services for initiation of cognitive behavioural therapy, interpersonal therapy, systemic family therapy or group therapy, depending on the case, applying protocols and scheduling consultations with the family doctor as indicated. If the patient does not improve with non-pharmacological treatments (such as exercise and healthy eating and psychotherapy) and pharmacological treatments (such as fluoxetine, sertraline or, in other cases, amitriptyline when the previous ones are not available), the patient is referred for evaluation by psychiatric services. Monitoring by psychological services and family medicine will continue while the patient is awaiting an appointment for second-level care.

However, many health professionals are unaware of the clinical guidelines published by the Ministry of Public Health and are not trained in the management of this type of mental disorder, which is a call to attention for universities that may not be giving importance to this situation in their classrooms. Another problem is that the public institution does not routinely train its doctors; in some places, they carry out online courses on the subject. Nursing staff are not in charge of identifying these disorders, so they are not trained to screen for these pathologies. The clinical guide is not used, either due to ignorance or lack of time because they only have 15 minutes for the consultation, which makes it difficult to detect people with depression and anxiety.

Health provision and education need to be coordinated. To ensure that depression and anxiety are adequately detected and managed, universities must prepare their future professionals to identify and treat these diseases in a timely manner. Both medical and nursing staff should be trained in the detection of these mental disorders.

REFERENCES

1. Cordero B, Bustamante JP, Guinad M. Nacionalidades y Pueblos Indígenas y políticas interculturales en Ecuador, Una mirada desde la Educación. 2010.
2. Educación Médica. Ecuador, entre los países con más casos de depresión en Latinoamérica. Ecuador. 2017;1. Accessed from: https://www.edicionmedica.ec/secciones/salud-publica/ecuador-entre-los-pa-ses-con-m-s-casos-de-depresi-n-en-latinoam-rica-89705
3. Our World in Data. Number of people with anxiety disorders, 1990 to 2019. 2019. p. 1.
4. Torres C, Otero P, Bustamante B, Blanco V, Díaz O, Vázquez FL. Mental health problems and related factors in ecuadorian college students. Int J Environ Res Public Health. 2017;14(5).
5. Sisa I, Vega R. Prevalencia de depresión en adultos mayores residentes en Ecuador y factores contribuyentes: un estudio poblacional. Rev Salud Publica. 2021;23(2):1–10.
6. Romero C, Saavedra M, Arévalo T, Molina J, Narea V View of Prevalencia de depresión y factores asociados, en estudiantes de Medicina, Cuenca - Ecuador, 2019.pdf. South Fla J Dev. 2022;3:1661–70. Accessed from: https://ojs.southfloridapublishing.com/ojs/index.php/jdev/article/view/1225/1009
7. Ministerio de Salud Pública. Diagnóstico y tratamiento del episodio depresivo y del trastorno depresivo recurrente en adultos. [Internet]. Msp. 2017. pp. 1–128.

CHAPTER 9

Depression and anxiety in primary care in North America

DOI: 10.1201/9781003391531-9

9.1 DEPRESSION AND ANXIETY IN CANADA

Alan Ng Cheng Hin

Mood and anxiety disorders are the most common mental health disorders seen in primary care in Canada. About three-quarters of Canadians who used health services for a mental illness annually consulted for mood and anxiety disorders. The highest prevalence was observed among those aged 30–54 years, followed by those 55 years and older.[1] In 2016, the largest relative increases in prevalence were found among children and youth (aged 5–14 years); in absolute terms, however, these increases were less than 1%.[1]

Anxiety is extremely common, with 2.6% of Canadians aged 15 years and older reporting symptoms within a 12-month period. Of these, 50% reported co-existing symptoms compatible with a major depressive episode. This is consistent with epidemiological studies using comparable methodology in the United States, Europe and Australia.[2]

Environmental and coping capacity factors are as important as genetics and neurochemistry in explaining the causes of depression and anxiety.[3] Adverse childhood events (ACEs) contribute significantly to a higher risk of depression later in life.[4] At-risk populations in Canada include a positive family history, female gender, lower socioeconomic status, indigenous (First Nations) status and accompanying chronic disease burden.[3]

Although the prevalence of depression and anxiety in Canada is significant, they remain challenging to diagnose and manage in primary care. Although the vast majority of mood disorders and anxiety present in primary care, the current understanding and clinical approach to them are often dominated by a model derived from psychiatry, where the focus is on psychological symptoms such as sadness or worry.[3] It is important to develop a model which is suitable for the primary care setting in order to approach depression and anxiety. Firstly, mental and medical disorders often coexist (comorbidity). Secondly depression and anxiety can present with chronic and disabling physical symptoms, with the physical symptoms often predominating and obscuring the psychological symptoms unless specifically sought out. Thirdly, depression and anxiety can present with chronic medically unexplained symptoms (MUS).[5]

The *Diagnostic and Statistical Manual of Mental Disorders* (DSM-5)[6] guides physicians in classifying depression and anxiety as distinct disease entities, the symptoms of which cut across most of clinical medicine. However, like other emotional experiences, the symptoms of anxiety and depression cannot be separated from the person experiencing them or their biological functions, and this requires a patient-centred approach from the treating clinician.[3,7]

Within Canada's public Medicare system, the primary care physician is the gatekeeper for initial contact with the health care system, and as such usually remains the de facto mental health provider.[8,9] Detection rates of mental disorders in primary care remain low for various reasons –limited time for appointments, a concentration on somatic presentations as the valid 'ticket of admission' and the stigma of mental illness, which provides challenges for patients to discuss their problems.[8]

Notwithstanding comorbidity with other chronic medical conditions and the association with medically unexplained symptoms, depression and anxiety also frequently coexist. Generalised anxiety disorder may precede a major depression, which adds to the diagnostic challenge.[3]

To diagnose anxiety or depression, attention to DSM-5 criteria provides guidance in order to identify specific conditions (major depressive disorder, generalised anxiety disorder, etc.) using targeted screening questions and screening tools such as the Patient Health Questionnaire (PHQ-9), Hamilton Depression Rating Scale (HAM-D), Beck Depression Inventory (BDI-II) and the General Anxiety Disorder Questionnaire (GAD-7).[8]

Although there is known to be under-recognition of depression and anxiety, the Canadian Task Force on Preventive Health Care (CTFPHC 2013) does not currently recommend screening for adults at average risk for depression or those who may be at increased risk.[10]

In Canada, treatment of depression and anxiety can be divided into two broad categories: Psychopharmacology (medication) and non-pharmaceutical interventions, which includes psychotherapy, psychoeducation and self-management. Using medication follows a step-wise approach, with first-line options followed by second-line options and then augmentation agents for resistant cases. For anxiety, antidepressants are the first-line medications for treatment, with anxiolytics being used for a brief duration, usually when antidepressants are being initiated and titrated upwards. For both depression and anxiety, augmentation agents include atypical antipsychotics, mood stabilisers and anticonvulsants.[8]

For mild to moderate depression, evidence-based psychotherapy is as effective as antidepressants. For patients with chronic, severe or treatment-resistant depression, or with a comorbid disorder such as anxiety or personality disorder, combined psychotherapy and medication works better than either treatment alone. Psychotherapy for depression includes cognitive behavioural therapy (CBT) and behavioural activation. For anxiety, CBT is the first-line psychotherapy with the best evidence base.[8,11] Treatment is individualised based upon acuity and severity of the condition, individual patient context and patient choice. With regard to the use of CBT, patient choice, motivation and insight are important considerations before using this option.[11]

Federal and provincial governments have been making clear efforts to increase access to mental health services.[12] However, the recent COVID-19 pandemic highlighted and augmented the morbidity and burden of depression and anxiety upon the general population and the health care system.[13,14] With the growing demand for mental health services in general and the associated high costs to Canada's health care system, there remains an urgent need for improved access and cost-efficient delivery in order to meet this need.

Other significant access challenges remain: Long wait times, shortage of accessible mental health professionals, lack of mental health service integration, culture and language barriers, concerns about stigma, inequities due to geography or demographics (e.g., youth, rural communities, and Indigenous populations) and cost of services not covered by private insurance plans.[12]

To improve detection and management of depression and anxiety in the primary care setting, a holistic and multipronged approach is required. This includes public awareness campaigns to reduce the stigma of mental health disorders. Integration and funding of community-based resources are necessary to decrease reliance on high-cost services like hospital-based emergency departments or psychiatrists, which contribute to access issues.[15] As the point of first contact, primary care providers need ongoing training on how to manage consultations with patients who present with symptoms which may not immediately point to a diagnosis of anxiety and depression. This requires attention to the biopsychosocial nature of anxiety and depression and building competency in patient-centred approaches to the consultation.[7] Primary care providers should develop a 'toolkit' of evidence-based approaches which includes office-based brief CBT techniques, behavioural activation and motivational interviewing, amongst others.[5,7,9,11]

REFERENCES

1. McRae L, O'Donnell S, Loukine L, Rancourt N, Pelletier C. Report summary - mood and anxiety disorders in Canada, 2016. Health Promot Chronic Dis Prev Can. 2016;36(12): 314–5. Available from: http://dx.doi.org/10.24095/hpcdp.36.12.05

2. Pelletier L, O'Donnell S, McRae L, Grenier J. The burden of generalized anxiety disorder in Canada. Health Promot Chronic Dis Prev Can. 2017;37(2):54–62. Available from: http://dx.doi.org/10.24095/hpcdp.37.2.04

3. Freeman TR. McWhinney's textbook of family medicine. 4th ed. New York, NY: Oxford University Press; 2016.

4. Afifi TO, MacMillan HL, Boyle M, Taillieu T, Cheung K, Sareen J. Child abuse and mental disorders in Canada. CMAJ. 2014;186(9):E324–E32. Available from: http://dx.doi.org/10.1503/cmaj.131792

5. Smith RC, D'Mello D, Osborn G, Freilich L, Dwamena F, Laird-Fick H. Essentials of psychiatry in primary care: behavioral health in the medical setting. Columbus, OH: McGraw-Hill Education; 2019

6. American Psychiatric Association. Diagnostic and statistical manual of mental disorders (DSM-5 (R)). 5th ed. Arlington, TX: American Psychiatric Association Publishing; 2013.

7. Stewart M, Brown JB, Weston WW, McWhinney IR, McWilliam CL, Freeman TR. Patient-centered medicine: Transforming the clinical method. 3rd ed. London, England: Radcliffe Publishing; 2013

8. Goldbloom D, Davine J, editors. Psychiatry in primary care: a concise Canadian pocket guide. Centre for Addiction and Mental Health. Toronto, Canada; 2019.

9. Stuart MR, Lieberman JA. The fifteen minute hour: efficient and effective patient-centered consultation skills, sixth edition. 6th ed. London, England: CRC Press; 2018.

10. Beck A, Hamel C, Thuku M, Esmaeilisaraji L, Bennett A, Shaver N, et al. Screening for depression among the general adult population and in women during pregnancy or the first-year postpartum: two systematic reviews to inform a guideline of the Canadian task force on preventive health care. Syst Rev. 2022;11(1):176. Available from: http://dx.doi.org/10.1186/s13643-022-02022-2

11. David L. Using CBT in general practice: the 10 minute consultation. 2nd ed. Bloxham, England: Scion Publishing; 2013.

12. Moroz N, Moroz I, D'Angelo MS. Mental health services in Canada: barriers and cost-effective solutions to increase access. Healthc Manage Forum. 2020;33(6):282–7. Available from: http://dx.doi.org/10.1177/0840470420933911

13. Dozois DJA, Mental Health Research Canada. Anxiety and depression in Canada during the COVID-19 pandemic: a national survey. Can Psychol. 2021;62(1):136–42. Available from: http://dx.doi.org/10.1037/cap0000251

14. Anxiety, feelings of depression and loneliness among Canadians spikes to highest levels since spring 2020. CAMH. [cited 2023 Jan 2]. Available from: https://www.camh.ca/en/camh-news-and-stories/anxiety-depression-loneliness-among-canadians-spikes-to-highest-levels

15. Ashcroft R, Menear M, Greenblatt A, Silveira J, Dahrouge S, Sunderji N, et al. Patient perspectives on quality of care for depression and anxiety in primary health care teams: a qualitative study. Health Expect. 2021;24(4):1168–77. Available from: http://dx.doi.org/10.1111/hex.13242

9.2 DEPRESSION AND ANXIETY IN THE UNITED STATES OF AMERICA

Lesca Hadley and Thomas Shima

Depression and anxiety are common conditions in the United States with potentially serious complications. These conditions are found in a wide range of patient populations with a predilection for certain groups. An estimated 18 million adults are affected by depression each year,[1] and 5–9 million adults are affected by generalised anxiety.[2] In 2017, 13% of US teens aged 12–17 (over 3 million) said they had experienced at least one major depressive episode or anxiety in the past year.[3]

A number of specific patient populations are at increased risk for both anxiety and depression. Adolescents and young adults (ages 12–24) have the highest percentages of both anxiety and depression.[3] Women are at higher risk for depression than men. In 2019, 21.8% of women experienced depression symptoms compared to 15.0% for men.[4] Women are also twice as likely to have anxiety than men.[1] Another at-risk population for anxiety and depression are patients with significant comorbidities such as diabetes, coronary artery disease, stroke, cancer and HIV.[5–9]

Depression and anxiety may manifest with similar symptoms. Adults with depression have episodes of sadness, loss of interest or pleasure in former activities, sleep disturbances, angry outbursts and feelings of worthlessness. In children and teens, symptoms of depression are similar, but with some differences such as excessive sleeping, refusal to attend school, poor grades and clinginess. Anxiety involves a heightened fear of things and loss of control. Adults and teens with anxiety are often on edge and overwhelmed with panic or a feeling of impending doom. They can also experience tremors, tachycardia, increased sweating and hyperventilation.

The primary care physician in the United States is often the clinician who makes the diagnosis of depression or anxiety. The *Diagnostic and Statistical Manual of Mental Disorders,* published by the American Psychiatric Association, provides specific diagnostic criteria for depression and anxiety. Several self-assessment screening tools are available to help the primary care physician make the diagnosis. For depression, these include the Patient Health Questionnaire-2 (PHQ-2) and the Patient Health Questionnaire-9 (PHQ-9). The PHQ-2 is a brief two-question test that enables the clinician to quickly assess whether further testing is needed. If the PHQ-2 test is positive, then the clinician should proceed to the PHQ-9 questionnaire for a more definitive diagnosis of depression. In the elderly, the Geriatric Depression Scale is recommended as a standardised screening tool.

Two self-assessment tools commonly used for anxiety are the Generalized Anxiety Disorder-7 (GAD-7) and the Screening for Child Anxiety Related

Disorders (SCARED). The SCARED tool is focused specifically on the child or teen patient. For children ages 8–11, it is recommended that the clinician explain all questions or have the child answer the questionnaire sitting with an adult in case they have any questions. Additionally, SCARED has a separate questionnaire that is completed by the parent. All these screening tools provide good evidence for making the diagnosis of depression or anxiety.

Most patients visit their primary care physician first for the treatment of anxiety and depression, although some patients may initially present to a psychiatrist.[10] Patients may also access help or information on their own for depression or anxiety through various phone hotlines and online websites.

Treatment with selective serotonin reuptake inhibitors and selective serotonin or norepinephrine reuptake inhibitors is first-line therapy for anxiety and depression. Benzodiazepines are not recommended for first-line therapy. Medications are recommended for 6–12 months following resolution of the depression and anxiety to prevent relapse. Psychotherapy, especially cognitive behavioural therapy, is recommended for anxiety and depression and is commonly used in combination with medications for treatment. If patients' symptoms do not respond to first-line treatments, primary care physicians will routinely refer the patients to psychiatrists. Often patients with depression and anxiety have comorbid substance abuse disorders which need professional treatment too.[11]

Stepped care approaches for mental health exist within some organisations and healthcare insurance plans. However, standardisation of a stepped approach across the country does not exist.[1] In recent years the emphasis on the detection and management of depression and anxiety in primary care has increased. National attention has been placed on mental health, with funding for treatment and education coming from the government as well as other sources.[12]

Physicians in primary care are trained to detect depression and anxiety in the outpatient setting. Nurses and medical assistants may collect information on depression and anxiety using screens under the direction of a physician. The detection and management of depression and anxiety still need to be improved. Studies show high rates of undetected depression and anxiety. The Centers for Disease Control and Prevention in the United States report that 1.2 million adults in the United States attempted suicide in 2020, with non-Hispanic American Indian and Alaskan natives disproportionally affected. Males accounted for approximately 80% of suicides, and the highest rate of suicide was in the elderly, in particular, people over the age of 85.[13]

Improving the detection and management of depression and anxiety will take a multifaceted approach. Education must occur on many levels. Depression often starts in the young, so educators who work with children need to be taught the signs and symptoms of depression and anxiety. Universities and workplaces need strategies to identify, support and treat their students and employees. The elderly need connection and support to adjust to life's changes, and their caregivers need to know the signs of a person at risk. Much of the country lacks adequate mental health services, so an emphasis must be placed on training the primary care workforce to combat depression and anxiety.[12] The workforce must then be attracted to work in places where they are most needed. Telehealth services are another way of extending the workforce into areas without access to mental health services.

REFERENCES

1. Kessler RC, Chiu WT, Demler O, Merikangas KR, Walters EE. Prevalence, severity, and comorbidity of 12-month DSM-IV disorders in the national comorbidity survey replication. Arch Gen Psychiatry. 2005;62(6):617–27.
2. Grant BF, Hasin DS, Stinson FS, Dawson DA, June Ruan W, Goldstein RB, Smith SM, Saha TD, Huang B. Prevalence, correlates, co-morbidity, and comparative disability of DSM-IV generalized anxiety disorder in the USA: results from the national epidemiologic survey on alcohol and related conditions. Psychol Med. 2005;35(12):1747–59.
3. Substance Abuse and Mental Health Services Administration. Key Substance Use and Mental Health Indicators in the United States: Results from the 2017 National Survey on Drug Use and Health (HHS Publication No. SMA 18-5068, NSDUH Series H-53). Rockville, MD: Center for Behavioral Health Statistics and Quality, Substance Abuse and Mental Health Services Administration. 2018. Retrieved from https://www.samhsa.gov/data/
4. National Center for Health Statistics. National Health Interview Survey. 2019.
5. Rabkin JG. HIV and depression: 2008 review and update. Curr HIV/AIDS Rep. 2008;5(4):163–71. Available from: http://dx.doi.org/10.1007/s11904-008-0025-1
6. Krebber AM, Buffart LM, Kleijn G, et al. Prevalence of depression in cancer patients: a meta-analysis of diagnostic interviews and self-report instruments. Psychooncology. 2014;23(2):121–30.
7. Walker J, Hansen CH, Martin P, et al. Prevalence, associations, and adequacy of treatment of major depression in patients with cancer: a cross-sectional analysis of routinely collected clinical data. Lancet Psychiatry. 2014 Oct;1(5):343–50. doi: 10.1016/S2215-0366(14)70313-X. Epub 2014 Aug 28.
8. Mitchell AJ, Chan M, Bhatti H, et al. Prevalence of depression, anxiety, and adjustment disorder in oncological, haematological, and palliative-care settings: a meta-analysis of 94 interview-based studies. Lancet Oncol. 2011;12(2):160–74.
9. Arun MPS, Bharath S, Pal P, Singh G. Relationship of depression, disability, and quality of life in Parkinson's disease: a hospital-based case-control study. Neurol India. 2011;59(2):185–89.
10. Haugh JA, et al. Acceptability of the stepped care model of depression treatment in primary care patients and providers. J Clin Psychol Med Settings. 2019;6(4):402–10.
11. DeGeorge KC, et al. Generalized anxiety disorder and panic disorder in adults. Am Fam Physician. 2022;106(2):157–64.
12. Crowley R, Kirschner N. The integration of care for mental health, substance abuse, and other behavioral health conditions into primary care: executive summary of an American college of physicians position paper. Ann Int Med. 2015;163(4):298–99.
13. Centers for Disease Control and Prevention. Suicide Data and Statistics CDC. https://www.cdc.gov/suicide/suicide-data-statistics.html (accessed Jan 2023).

CHAPTER 10

Depression and anxiety in primary care in South Asia

DOI: 10.1201/9781003391531-10

10.1 DEPRESSION AND ANXIETY IN NEPAL

Pramendra Prasad Gupta

In Nepal, the prevalence of depressive symptoms has been reported to range from 27% to 76%.[1-3] The limited studies on anxiety have estimated the proportion of symptoms to range from 10% to 57%.[3-6] In adolescents, studies have found that male gender, staying away from home, grade and stream of study, academic performance, examination-related issues and cyber bullying are all linked with depression. Likewise, gender, grade of students and type of school (i.e., public or private), family type, not living with parents, educational level of parents and high educational stress have been found to be determinants of anxiety.[7,8]

Depression may manifest as feelings of sadness, tearfulness, emptiness or hopelessness, along with angry outbursts, irritability or frustration, even over small matters. Other symptoms include loss of interest or pleasure in most or all normal activities and sleep disturbances, including insomnia or sleeping too much. Anxiety manifests as feeling tense, nervous or unable to relax, having a sense of dread or fear while going in a crowd, loss of appetite and sleep, palpitation, sweating or feeling like the world is speeding up or slowing down. In Nepal, the Patient Health Questionnaire 9-item (PHQ-9) tool may be used to diagnose depression, and *Diagnostic and Statistical Manual of Mental Disorders, Fourth Edition* (DSM-IV) criteria may be used for both depression and anxiety.

While mental health services are supposed to be included among the basic health services expected to be delivered in primary health care (PHC) in Nepal, there is little evidence that these services are delivered in PHC settings in practice. The Management Division, a section of the Department of Health Services, mental hospitals and some non-governmental organisations (NGOs) have taken the initiative to train PHC workers in a few districts.[9] However, the lack of refresher training and non-availability of essential psychotropic medicines has meant that, despite the training provided, there continues to be a lack of availability of mental health services on a regular basis. Two psychotropic medications, phenobarbitone and amitriptyline, are available in PHC centres and, more erratically, at the Health Post level, but no psychotropic medicines are available at the Sub-Health Post level. No counselling or psychotherapeutic services are available through the PHC system. Due to the lack of clear referral mechanisms from primary to tertiary care, people with mental illness are not being identified or treated effectively, even in the health facilities where there are trained health workers. No standardised training manuals, screening tools or guidelines are available, particularly for the training of PHC workers in the detection, diagnosis and treatment of common and severe mental disorders.[9]

Despite this bleak mental health situation, Nepal has made significant improvements in recent years, in comparison to a situation analysis using the World Health Organization Assessment Instrument for Mental Health Systems (WHO-AIMS) in 2006.[10] For example, the total number of psychiatrists has increased considerably. The number of mental health beds was less than 1 (0.8) per 100,000 population[10] and has now increased to 1.5 per 100,000 population. The involvement of user groups in mental health care, prevention and advocacy has become more established, and two national-level organisations led by service users have been instituted. Community-based mental health programmes have been initiated in a few districts by both the government and NGOs.[11,12] In recent years, some initiatives have been taken to include mental health in national health priorities. For example, mental health has been included in the second health-sector support programme (NHSSP-II), 'one stop' crisis centres have been established and psychosocial and mental health has been included in national minimum standards and standard operating procedures for the care and protection of survivors of trafficking.[13] Additionally, mental health and psychosocial components in the protection and care for children affected by HIV/AIDS[14] and the provision of psychotropic medicines in the revised drug lists are key policy-level initiatives in mental health and psychosocial care.[9]

Recently, a consortium of research institutions and ministries of health in five countries in Asia and Africa (India, Nepal, South Africa, Ethiopia and Uganda), with partners in the United Kingdom and the WHO, has established the PRogramme for Improving Mental health carE (PRIME) to study the implementation and scaling up of treatment programmes for priority mental disorders in primary and maternal health care contexts.[9]

In future, to strengthen mental health services, it will be better to coordinate mental health activities and issues with the government at the central and district level, if a separate mental health unit were to be established in the Ministry of Health and Population. The situation would also be improved by training of health care providers at the PHC level and development of a mid-level mental health and psychosocial cadre within the PHC system. An efficient referral mechanism should be established to provide specialist mental health services to people with severe mental disorders where no mental health services are currently available. NGOs can play an important role in developing and delivering models for more innovative services, supporting government initiatives and building capacity.

REFERENCES

1. Bhattarai D, Shrestha N, Paudel S. Prevalence and factors associated with depression among higher secondary school adolescents of Pokhara Metropolitan, Nepal: a cross-sectional study. BMJ Open. 2020;10:e044042. pmid:33384401

2. Gautam P, Dahal M, Ghimire H, Chapagain S, Baral K, Acharya R, et al. Depression among adolescents of rural Nepal: a community-based study. Depress Res Treat. 2021;2021. pmid:33628501

3. Bhandari M. Anxiety and depression among adolescent students at higher secondary school. BIBECHANA. 2016;14:113–29. doi: 10.3126/bibechana.v14i0.16019

4. Bhandari K, Adhikari C. Prevalence and factors associated with anxiety disorder among secondary school adolescents of Dang district, Nepal. J Gandaki Med Coll Nepal. 2015 [cited 2 Jan 2022] 8:53–56.

5. Sharma P, Choulagai B. Stress, Anxiety, and Depression Among Adolescent Students of Public Schools in Kathmandu. [cited 19 Mar 2022]. Available from: www.jiom.com.np

6. Nepal Health Research Council. National Mental Health Survey, Nepal-2020. In: Nepal Health Research Council. 2020 pp. 1–4. Available from: http://nhrc.gov.np/projects/nepal-mental-health-survey-2017-2018/

7. Kumar KS, Akoijam BS. Depression, anxiety and stress among higher secondary school students of Imphal, Manipur. Indian J Community Med. 2017;42:94. pmid:28553025

8. Karki A, Thapa B, Pradhan PMS, Basel P. Depression, anxiety and stress among high school students: a cross-sectional study in an urban municipality of Kathmandu, Nepal. PLoS Glob Public Health. 2022;2(5):e0000516. doi: 10.1371/journal.pgph.0000516

9. Luitel NP, Jordans MJ, Adhikari A, Upadhaya N, Hanlon C, Lund C, Komproe IH. Mental health care in Nepal: current situation and challenges for development of a district mental health care plan. Confl Health. 2015 Feb 6;9:3. doi: 10.1186/s13031-014-0030-5

10. WHO. WHO-AIMS Report on Mental Health System in Nepal. Kathmandu: World Health Organization and Ministry of Health; 2006.

11. Upadhyaya K, Nakarmi B, Prajapati B, Timilsina M. Morbidity profile of patients attending the centers for mental health service provided jointly by the government of Nepal and community mental health service of community mental health and counseling-Nepal (CMC-Nepal). J Psychiatrists' Assoc Nepal. 2013;2(1):14–9.

12. Raja S, Underhill C, Shrestha P, Sunder U, Mannarath S, Wood SK, et al. Integrating mental health and development: a case study of the basic needs model in Nepal. PLoS Med. 2012;9(7):e1001261. doi: 10.1371/journal.pmed.1001261.

13. Ministry of Women, Children and Social Welfare. National Minimum Standard for the Care and Protection of Victims/Survivors of Trafficking in Persons. Kathmandu: MWCSW. 2012.

14. Ministry of Health and Population. Mainstreaming Psychosocial Care in the Existing Health Care System for Children Affected by AIDS MoHP Kathmandu. 2012.

10.2 DEPRESSION AND ANXIETY IN PAKISTAN

Saniya Sabzwari

Different prevalence studies conducted in Pakistan cite high rates of depression and anxiety that range from 30% to 60%.[1-3] Reasons for this higher-than-average prevalence are multiple. Pakistan has a high burden of infectious and non-communicable diseases. Chronic infectious diseases like tuberculosis have been associated with an increased risk of depression and anxiety.[4] A recent meta-analysis explored the link between non-communicable disease burden and anxiety and depression, and diabetic patients' reported anxiety ranged from 12% to more than 50%.[5] Women and young people are at greater risk for anxiety and depression. For women, additional risk factors include family structure and perinatal health.[1,6,7] A systematic review identified a more than 40% prevalence of depression and anxiety among university students, a large proportion with their first episode before the age of 20.[8] Adolescents are also at greater risk largely due to socioeconomic factors.[9] A more recent survey that looked at anxiety and depression due to the pandemic lockdown cited higher rates, mostly in younger adults. Older individuals are also at high risk in a recent community-based study, where more than 50% of older adults had a positive PHQ-2.[10]

In Pakistan depression and anxiety most commonly manifest as somatic symptoms which are often multiple and of a chronic nature not responding to usual care. The most common symptoms are fatigue, body aches, headaches, dizziness and palpitations. On occasion patients directly report low mood and symptoms of constant worry or situational stress.

Various tools are available for screening and diagnosing depression and anxiety in Pakistan. The PHQ-2 has become the universal screening tool for depression, used to screen patients presenting with multiple unexplained somatic complaints, low mood or decline in functionality. When the PHQ-2 is positive, then the PHQ-9 is used to determine the severity of depression. There is a validated Urdu (local language) version of PHQ-9 which makes it a useful tool.[11] A locally developed and validated tool the Aga Khan University Anxiety and Depression Scale (AKUADS) for diagnosis of depression and anxiety in various out-patient and community settings is also available.[12] The screening tool most used for anxiety is the Generalized Anxiety Disorder 7-item scale (GAD-7), which has also been translated and validated in Pakistan.[13] While these tools are freely available and use has been validated via local research, diagnosis in clinical practice is largely based on clinical symptoms after ruling out physical causes. Use of validated tools is varied, and criteria for screening are non-uniform.

No national guidelines exist for the management of depression and anxiety; hence, the management approaches are diverse, and no algorithmic approach is used. Primary care largely exists outside the realm of academic institutions – independent practitioners in private practice serving urban and rural areas – and therefore approaches differ. Moreover, patients' perceptions and stigma related to mental health often play a major role in the management.[14] Patients very often seek care from faith healers and hesitate to take medications that specifically target their depression or anxiety.[15] Physician perceptions and understanding of common mental health issues also influence care.[16] In one study benzodiazepines were cited as the mainstay of treatment by general practitioners,[17] and knowledge about common pharmacological agents was cited as low in another.[18]

Non-pharmacological interventions like psychotherapy play a limited role, largely due to a small number of providers; a pay-out-of-pocket health care system; and reluctance of patients to use counselling services due to perceived ineffectiveness, stigma and other cultural beliefs.[19] Guideline development for depression and anxiety for primary care providers is currently underway. Its completion and dissemination should improve the management approach to these disorders.

Detection and management of depression and anxiety is not given a priority in our country for multiple reasons. There are approximately 500 psychiatrists serving a population of more than 200 million. General practitioners and non-psychiatric specialists do not receive basic mental health education during their training, and there exists a strong stigma towards mental illness along with poor advocacy. Only a small number of physicians, nurses and community health workers through various academic and private institutions have received any training in this area.[20]

Diagnosis and management of depression and anxiety need to be an integral part of primary care. Introduction to these common mental health conditions should start at an undergraduate level in medical schools across Pakistan to sensitize future physicians. Development of a national guideline for screening and treatment will streamline and standardise care of patients. Improving mental health literacy and increasing awareness at multiple levels of providers may improve care provision for these conditions.

REFERENCES

1. Muhammad Gadit AA, Mugford G. Prevalence of depression among households in three capital cities of Pakistan: need to revise the mental health policy. PLoS ONE. 2007;2(2):e209.
2. Ahmed B, Enam SF, Iqbal Z, et al. Depression and anxiety: a snapshot of the situation in Pakistan. Int J Neurosci Behav Sci. 2016;4(2):32.
3. Uphoff EP, Newbould L, Walker I, et al. A systematic review and meta-analysis of the prevalence of common mental disorders in people with non-communicable diseases in Bangladesh, India, and Pakistan. J Glob Health. 2019;9(2).

4. Husain MO, Dearman SP, Chaudhry IB, et al. The relationship between anxiety, depression and illness perception in tuberculosis patients in Pakistan. Clin Pract Epidemiology Ment Health. 2008;4(1):1–5.
5. Farooq S, Khan T, Zaheer S, et al. Prevalence of anxiety and depressive symptoms and their association with multimorbidity and demographic factors: a community-based, cross-sectional survey in Karachi, Pakistan. BMJ Open. 2019;9(11):e029315.
6. Atif M, Halaki M, Raynes-Greenow C, et al. Perinatal depression in Pakistan: a systematic review and meta-analysis. Birth. 2021;48(2):149–63.
7. Insan N, Weke A, Forrest S, et al. Social determinants of antenatal depression and anxiety among women in South Asia: a systematic review & meta-analysis. PLoS ONE 2022;17(2):e0263760.
8. Khan MN, Akhtar P, Ijaz S, et al. Prevalence of depressive symptoms among university students in Pakistan: a systematic review and meta-analysis. Front Public Health. 2021;8:603357.
9. Khalid A, Qadir F, Chan SW, et al. Adolescents' mental health and well-being in developing countries: a cross-sectional survey from Pakistan. J Ment Health. 2019;28(4):389–96.
10. Sabzwari SR, Iqbal R, Fatmi Z, et al. Factors associated with geriatric morbidity and impairment in a megacity of Pakistan. PLoS ONE. 2019;14(6):e0218872.
11. Ahmad S, Hussain S, Akhtar F, et al. Urdu translation and validation of PHQ-9, a reliable identification, severity and treatment outcome tool for depression. J Pak Med Assoc. 2018;68(8):1166–70.
12. Ali BS, Reza H, Khan MM, et al. Development of an indigenous screening instrument in Pakistan: the aga khan university anxiety and depression scale. J Pak Med Assoc. 1998;48(9):261.
13. Ahmad S, Hussain S, Shah FS, et al. Urdu translation and validation of GAD-7: a screening and rating tool for anxiety symptoms in primary health care. J Pak Med Assoc. 2017;67(10):1536–40.
14. Nisar M, Mohammad RM, Fatima S, et al. Perceptions pertaining to clinical depression in Karachi, Pakistan. Cureus. 2019;11(7).
15. Choudhry FR, Khan N, Munawar K. Barriers and facilitators to mental health care: a systematic review in Pakistan. Int J Ment Health. 2021:1–39.
16. Afridi MI, Dars JA, Lal C, et al. The perspective of general practitioners about mental illness: a cross-sectional observational study from a tertiary care centre, Pakistan. Perspective. 2021;33(43B).
17. Naqvi H, Sabzwari S, Hussain S, et al. General practitioners' awareness and management of common psychiatric disorders: a community-based survey from Karachi, Pakistan. East Mediterr Health J. 2012;18(5):446–53.
18. Rahman T, Amjad T, Minhas FA, et al. Integration of mental health into primary healthcare-a challenge for primary care physicians. Pak Armed Forces Med J. 2019;69.
19. Husain W. Barriers in seeking psychological help: public perception in Pakistan. Community Ment Health l. 2020;56(1):75–78.
20. Najam S, Chachar AS, Mian A. The mhgap; will it bridge the mental health treatment gap in Pakistan? Pak J of Neurol Sci. 2019;14(2):28–33.

CHAPTER 11

Depression and anxiety in migrant, refugee and war-zone populations

DOI: 10.1201/9781003391531-11

11.1 SCREENING OF MIGRANTS IN CANADA

David Ponka

Canada aims to welcome 465,000 new immigrants in 2023, 485,000 in 2024 and 500,000 in 2025.[1] This continues a tradition of openness in a vast, sparsely populated country to sustain growth and pluralism. A significant proportion of these migrants (projected to increase to over 70,000 per annum) are refugees fleeing persecution or violence under the protection of the Geneva Convention. The clinician must thus develop an understanding of each migrant's journey and how it affects the approach to care, including mental health screening.

Efforts to coordinate immigrant and refugee screening of mental health conditions are tied to several common Canadian health care challenges. These include a devolved health system to the provincial level, a highly heterogeneous primary care sector, lack of system integration including information systems, and inadequate mental health services for all Canadians. Despite this, Canadian society continues to value immigration, and federal protections and supports are in place to provide funding for health services for migrants as they await provincial-level supports.

This Interim Federal Health Programme (IFHP) contains provisions for mental health supports that, in some cases, exceed those of provincial systems, including psychological counselling. When the IFHP has been from time to time challenged in the political arena, Canadian physicians and health care supports have rallied around it, and this has led to content expertise and a Canadian Collaboration for Immigrant and Refugee Health (CCIRH).

THE BURDEN OF MENTAL HEALTH

The burden of mental health illness amongst immigrants to Canada follows that of all illness: Immigrants arrive to Canada healthier than the Canadian average, but this advantage diminishes and, in some cases, reverses over time. A recent study linking provincial records to national census data[2] found that while mood disorders were the leading cause of hospitalisations amongst all Canadians and female Canadian immigrants, psychotic disorders were more important amongst immigrant males. Anxiety disorders were a much less important cause of hospitalisation for all Canadians, perhaps reflecting disease that is less severe but nonetheless an important burden in the community. Specifically, post-traumatic stress disorders (PTSDs) have been highlighted in recent refugee waves from war-torn countries, including from Afghanistan, the Yazidi movement related to the Daesh insurgency in Iraq (including PTSD related to a high burden of gender-based violence), Syria and, more recently Ukraine.

In a review in the *Canadian Medical Association Journal* in 2011,[3] the CCIRH used the Delphi method to ask health care providers to rank the top 20 health conditions of greatest concern to immigrants and refugees coming to Canada. Again, depression and PTSD featured highly in the final ranking. Clinical experience also suggests that the incidence of complex post-traumatic stress disorder (cPTSD) is rising.[4] cPTSD can be a result of repeated, severe exposure to trauma affecting personal safety and can lead to a presentation akin to developmental delay in children, with emotional autoregulation being particularly affected. Management requires a team-based approach with integrated community services. It is also interesting to note that severe cPTSD can sometimes mimic psychosis.

THE CASE FOR SCREENING FOR DEPRESSION AND PTSD

Based on such considerations, it is possible to formulate a risk assessment[5] to help determine when to screen for mental health concerns in immigrant populations, namely depression and PTSD/severe anxiety. Forced migration, especially in the face of trauma threatening personal or family safety, as well as family separation, carries the highest risk. It is important to weigh the benefits of screening against the possible risks, including re-traumatisation, especially when trust and safety have not yet been established in the clinical setting. It is also important to have integrated and appropriate services available for individuals who screen positive.

The Canadian Immigration Medical Examination (IME) is administered pre-arrival, typically overseas, and is meant to ensure public safety. The IME simply asks: 'Have you ever had anxiety, depression or nervous problems requiring treatment?' Answers to this question are not available to the eventual treating team due to privacy reasons and limitations of data continuity between pre-arrival and post-arrival, as well as between federal and provincial jurisdictions.

It is very important to remember the difference between screening and case-finding. Even when universal screening is not advised, responding to obvious distress and symptomatology always is. Table 11.1 summarises the expert recommendations of the CCIRH on screening for depression and PTSD in migrants coming to Canada.[3]

TABLE 11.1 Recommendations from the Canadian Collaboration for Immigrant and Refugee Health (CCIRH) for depression[3]

If an integrated treatment programme is available, screen adults for depression using a systematic clinical inquiry or validated patient health questionnaire (PHQ-9 or equivalent).
Link suspected cases of depression with an integrated treatment programme and case management or mental health care.
Recommendations from CCIRH: post-traumatic stress disorder
Do not conduct routine screening for exposure to traumatic events, because pushing for disclosure of traumatic events in well-functioning individuals may result in more harm than good.
Be alert for signs and symptoms of post-traumatic stress disorder, especially in the context of unexplained somatic symptoms, sleep disorders or mental health disorders such as depression or panic disorder, and perform clinical assessment as needed to address functional impairment.

CHOICE OF INSTRUMENT

A Canadian team recently[6] completed a scoping review of screening instruments in the international literature. The team examined evidence for 85 screening instruments and found no consensus regarding the best mental health screening tool to be applied in the context of resettlement.

In the face of this uncertainty, the clinician should be compelled to use evidence-based screening tools for the general population in a culturally sensitive and trauma-informed manner.[7] In a busy setting, this can be done using sequential screening,[8] using validated tools such as the Patient Health Questionnaire 2-item scale (PHQ-2) (Table 11.2)[9] and followed by the PHQ-9 if necessary to detect depression. The number needed to screen using the PHQ-9 to prevent one person with persistent depression is only 18 amongst migrants coming to Canada.[3]

Although routine screening for PTSD in most settings is not advised, it is useful to review the relevant symptomatology for both PTSD and cPTSD (Table 11.3).

The scoping review is useful to point to screening instruments for particular clinical circumstances, including for survivors of torture.[10] It also points to instruments that are more appropriate to be administered by lay people and self-administered, including using digital technologies when literacy levels allow.[11] It is important not to miss the chance for screening because a particular screening instrument could not be identified or located due to time, technological or proprietary reasons.

TABLE 11.2 PHQ-2 instrument with validity measures in a general population[9]

Over the **last 2 weeks**, how often have you been bothered by the following problems?
Not at all (0 points); several days (1 point); more than half the days (2 points); nearly every day (3 points)

1. Little interest or pleasure in doing things
2. Feeling down, depressed or hopeless

Interpretation:

If the score is 3 or greater, major depressive disorder is more likely (see validity information below)
Patients who screen positive should be further evaluated with the PHQ-9, other diagnostic instruments or direct interview to determine whether they meet criteria for a depressive disorder.

PHQ-2 score	Sensitivity	Specificity
1	97.6	59.2
2	92.7	73.7
3	82.9	90.0
4	73.2	93.3
5	53.7	96.8
6	26.8	99.4

TABLE 11.3 Domains of enquiry in PTSD and complex PTSD

Four Areas of Disturbance in PTSD	1. Intrusive memories
	2. Avoidance
	3. Negative changes in thinking or mood, depression
	4. Hypervigilance
Additional Disturbances in cPTSD	1. Emotional regulation
	2. Self-identity
	3. Relational capacities

CULTURAL AND TRAUMA-INFORMED CARE

Canada's multicultural context is a good platform for developing an expertise in culturally appropriate and trauma-informed care. These values need to underpin programme development and delivery in busy clinical settings.

While families can be seen together when appropriate, translators should never be family members for confidentiality reasons save in the direst emergencies. Working effectively and in a patient-centred manner through translators takes training and experience. For example, one should always be seated facing the patient to observe body language and pause frequently to be able to understand verbal nuance through the translator.

Canada's multicultural context has helped develop expertise in culture-bound syndromes which reflect pluralism and diversity.[12] We have found that these are especially important coming from regions where mental illness faces important stigma. Knowledge of these specific patterns will help avoid over-investigation and lead to more timely mental health screening in view of earlier and more effective treatment. Trauma-informed approaches emphasise to first establish safety and trust with the provider and clinical milieu. This is a prerequisite to screening for mental health illness to avoid perpetuating or even amplifying the effect of past distress.

THE NEED TO LINK TO TREATMENT

Routine universal screening can cause harm if access to treatments that the patient can trust is lacking. Such trust is best established in integrated and stepped programmes, especially those that respond to the specific needs of patients from different backgrounds.[13] An integrated approach is one where referrals to allied health professionals and specialists occur in an environment already familiar to the patient, whereas a stepped approach is one that is appropriate for the symptomatology of the patient and can be escalated if necessary. Universal screening, especially of PTSD, should only occur when and where treatment can be offered.

Migrants from certain cultures may be more comfortable with group therapy than may be typical for other Canadian populations.

Several more recent, non-pharmacological clinical modalities have been studied amongst trauma victims, including refugees. Eye-movement desensitisation and reprocessing (EMDR) is a fascinating advance that uses highly specialised and structured interventions that involve bilateral stimulation (usually eye movements) while the patient is briefly focused on a trauma memory. It has been shown, including through neuro-imaging, to reduce the vividness of recall and emotion associated with trauma.

The process of narrative exposure therapy (NET) is perhaps more accessible. It can be used in primary care with physical props such as a string, stones and flowers or other culturally appropriate symbols. Actively playing out and reciting both negative and positive experiences in the context of the patient's whole life (represented by a long string purposefully extended beyond current events) also modulates harmful neural patterns that otherwise can remain latent (Figure 11.1).[14]

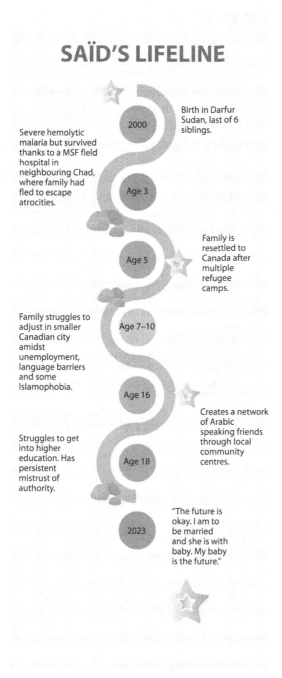

FIGURE 11.1 Narrative exposure therapy: an example of a lifeline.[14]

SCREENING IN CONTEXT

More recently, the COVID-19 pandemic both increased the need for and challenged the access to mental health services.[15,16] This crisis presents an opportunity to integrate specialised psychiatric services into primary care using a shared mental health approach.[17] Such approaches are best achieved through long-term relationships in a patient medical home model, engendering the trust[18] necessary to permit effective, and safe, mental health screening. Integrated community-based approaches are also crucial to link clinical and social services.

In the end, migration is a human transition amongst other life events that primary care providers have the merits to look after well. Just like during birth, hospitalisation or death, transitions require good communication skills, involvement of the family and awareness of the greater patient context.

REFERENCES

1. Government of Canada. Notice – Supplementary Information for the 2023–2025 Immigration Levels Plan - Canada.ca. Available from: https://www.canada.ca/en/immigration-refugees-citizenship/news/notices/supplementary-immigration-levels-2023-2025.html.
2. Grundy A et al. Mental health and neurocognitive disorders-related hospitalization rates in immigrants and Canadian-born population: a linkage study. Can J Public Health. 2023;114:692–704.
3. Pottie K et al. Evidence-based clinical guidelines for immigrants and refugees. CMAJ. 2011;183:E824–925.
4. Cyr G, Godbout N, Cloitre M, Bélanger C. Distinguishing among symptoms of posttraumatic stress disorder, complex posttraumatic stress disorder, and borderline personality disorder in a community sample of women. J Trauma Stress. 2022;35:186–96.
5. Wilkinson L, Ponka D. Mental health of immigrants and refugees in Canada. In Migration, Health and Survival: International Perspective. Edward Elgar Publishing: 2017, pp. 88–109. doi: 10.4337/9781785365973.00011
6. Magwood O et al. Mental health screening approaches for resettling refugees and asylum seekers: a scoping review. Int J Environ Res Public Health. 2022;19:3549.
7. Kirmayer LJ et al. Common mental health problems in immigrants and refugees: general approach in primary care. CMAJ. 2011;183:E959–E967.
8. Poole DN et al. Sequential screening for depression in humanitarian emergencies: a validation study of the patient health questionnaire among Syrian refugees. Ann Gen Psychiatry. 2020;19:5.
9. Kroenke K, Spitzer RL, Williams JBW. The patient health questionnaire-2: validity of a two-item depression screener. Med Care. 2003;41:1284–92.
10. Mewes R, Friele B, Bloemen E. Validation of the protect questionnaire: a tool to detect mental health problems in asylum seekers by non-health professionals. Torture. 2018;28:56–71.
11. Bjärtå A, Leiler A, Ekdahl J, Wasteson E. Assessing severity of psychological distress among refugees with the refugee health screener, 13-item version. J Nerv Ment Dis. 2018;206:834–39.
12. Kirmayer LJ, Sartorius N. Cultural models and somatic syndromes. Psychosom Med. 2007;69:832–40.

13. Ementalhealth. Specific Groups and Populations. Toronto, ON: Mental Health Services, Help and Support: eMentalHealth.ca. Available from: https://www.ementalhealth.ca/Toronto/Specific-Groups-and-Populations/index.php?m=heading&ID=126.
14. Ponka D. Little Seïd. Open Medicine. 2007;1:e164.
15. Benjamen J et al. Access to refugee and migrant mental health care services during the first six months of the covid-19 pandemic: a Canadian refugee clinician survey. Int J Environ Res Public Health. 2021;18:52–66.
16. Brickhill-Atkinson M, Hauck FR. Impact of COVID-19 on resettled refugees. Prim Care. 2021;48:57–66.
17. Rockman, P, Salach, L, Gotlib, D, Cord, M, Turner, T. Shared mental health care. Model for supporting and mentoring family physicians. Can Fam Physician. 2004;50:397–402.
18. Damji, AN et al. Trust as the foundation: thoughts on the Starfield principles in Canada and Brazil. Can Fam Physician. 2018;64:811–15.

11.2 MENTAL HEALTH SCREENING OF SYRIAN, IRAQI, AFGHAN AND OTHER REFUGEES AWAITING MIGRATION FROM TÜRKIYE TO THE UNITED STATES

Mehmet Ungan and Aysegul Cömert

INTRODUCTION

Drawing on data from the Internal Displacement Monitoring Centre, the United Nations High Commissioner for Refugees (UNHCR) estimates that global forced displacement reached 103 million in mid-2022, of whom 53.2 million were internally displaced people, 4.9 million were asylum-seekers and 5.3 million were other people in need of international protection. The UNHCR estimates that refugee numbers reached 32.5 million in mid-2022.[1,2]

Millions of Syrians (50% of refugees are Syrian), and now Ukrainians, have been displaced, with further displacement elsewhere in 2022. This means that 1 in every 78 people on earth has been forced to flee – a dramatic milestone that few would have expected a decade ago.

Refugees are defined narrowly by the Refugee Convention as individuals who have been forcibly displaced outside their native countries. Hundreds of millions of forced displaced people could be at excess risk of psychiatric morbidity. The relevant epidemiological evidence is, however, generally sparse, scattered and apparently conflicting. Türkiye hosts the largest number of refugees, with 3.7 million people officially registered. No one really knows the real numbers, as many are not registered or now have Turkish citizenship. The population of Türkiye is 85 million, roughly 10% of whom are migrants. Some of them are aiming to migrate to the United States of America. Immigrant medicals are performed in Ankara, and refugee medicals are performed in Istanbul.

MENTAL HEALTH ISSUES IN REFUGEES AND MIGRANTS

A screening programme for migrants to the United States is run through the Centers for Disease Control and Prevention's (CDC's) Division of Global Migration and Quarantine, Quality Assessment Program (QAP) of the United States. Panel physicians (PPs) are medically trained on technical instructions (TIs), are licensed and experienced general practitioners/family doctors (GPs/FDs) practising overseas and are authorised by the local US embassy or consulate under approval of the CDC. More than 760 GPs/FDs worldwide are PPs, performing overseas pre-departure medical examinations in accordance with requirements of the TIs. Two main groups are screened in primary care panel practices: Immigrants and refugees. Screening consists of physical and mental examination and laboratory tests including urinary drug screening when necessary. Mental evaluation is routine during the consultation, and short mental screening tests in applicants' languages are also used, such as the PHQ-9 depression scale, Generalized Anxiety Disorder (GAD) and State/Trait Anxiety Inventory anxiety tests and PTSD-4 for post-traumatic stress disorder. Any suspected harmful behaviour or substance use is referred to panel psychiatrists who have specific CDC TI training. A diagnosis of harmful behaviour or substance use is an inadmissible condition named as Class A. Other mental conditions usually require a follow-up before and/or after arrival to the United States, which is noted in the final report.

Refugees may present differently in primary care, because they have been forcibly displaced, not moving from choice. Unlike refugees, immigrants are motivated to leave their native countries for a variety of reasons, including a desire like marriage, a fiancée, economic prosperity, family reunification, escaping conflict or natural disaster or simply the wish to change one's surroundings. Migrants seen in PP practices usually tend to hide their mental conditions, do not seek help and generally are more mentally healthy, as they have chosen to live in another country. Diagnostic tools or *Diagnostic and Statistical Manual of Mental Disorders, Fifth Edition* (DSM-V) guidelines are rarely applied to immigrants, as they do not seek any help, and the guidelines usually used are those that are developed for routine clinical practice. It is for the primary care provider who cares for immigrants to identify those who need help but are not asking for it.

Whatever the reason, GPs/FDs should pay special attention to the mental condition of migrants, but especially of refugees, as they usually need help from outside their home countries and suffer (or fear) persecution on account of race, religion, nationality or political opinion; because they are a member of a persecuted social category of persons; or because they are fleeing a war.

As primary care providers, we experience that refugees seek help and try to shorten the waiting period here in Türkiye where they are temporary visitors, or tend to hide culturally unacceptable things that happened in their history. A GP/FD must be careful about the reliability of history. A large percentage of refugees may develop symptoms of PTSD or depression. These long-term mental problems can severely impede the functionality of the person in everyday situations; it makes matters even worse for displaced persons who are confronted with a new environment and challenging situations. Among other symptoms, PTSD involves anxiety, over-alertness, sleeplessness, chronic fatigue syndrome, motor difficulties, failing short-term memory, amnesia, nightmares and sleep paralysis. Depression is also characteristic for PTSD patients and may occur without accompanying PTSD.

CLASS A AND CLASS B MENTAL CONDITIONS

Final diagnosis of the mental condition in detail is not our aim in primary care, but rather identifying the presence of any harmful behaviour or potentially harmful conditions and preventing harm. A patient with a disease associated with any harmful behaviour (Class A) cannot migrate. Those requiring only follow-up and treatment but who can travel are instructed to have a follow-up – these are Class B mental conditions. We have checked our data in hand from May 2014 to March 2022 and tried to share any differences between the mental disorder prevalence of refugees and immigrants of the same nationality (i.e., Iran) living in Türkiye in the same time period.

We have extracted the Class B and Class A mental classifications from our software both for refugees and also for the immigrants. The data were searched for both refugees and immigrants between May 2014 and November 2022 (past eight years), and 24,224 immigrants and 25,582 refugees (total of 49806) were included.

As shown in Table 11.4, Iranian, Iraqi, Afghan and Syrian are the major nationalities screened as immigrants and refugees. The Iranian population is high in immigrants, whereas the Iraqi population was highest among refugees.

As others are not well comparable due to small sample sizes, we have checked the prevalence of mental condition only between the refugees and immigrants, and there was a statistically significant difference between the prevalence of mental condition of the two migrant groups of the Iranian and Afghan nationalities ($p < 0.05$). Afghan refugees have a significantly higher mental condition prevalence (19.1%) compared with the other nationalities ($p > 0.05$). The prevalence in Afghan refugees (22.1%) is considerably higher than in Afghan immigrants (4.1%). One in five of the Afghans in the sample had at least one mental condition.

When we look at the diagnostic distribution according to DSM-V, the immigrants are more likely to have mental conditions such as anxiety or minor depressive disorders, whereas the refugees may have PTSD or major depression, congenital or acquired neurological defects and other serious conditions.

A review by the World Health Organization (WHO) estimates the point prevalence of mental disorders as around 8–28% (22%).[3] However, there is considerable heterogeneity among studies in the literature, with variability in results due potentially to methodological factors such as differences in assessment tools and sampling, studies using clinical interviews (instead of self-report instruments), random sampling and larger sample sizes report- ing lower rates of mental disorders. Other differences in refugee populations in terms of trauma exposure, migration difficulties and living conditions in host countries may explain heterogeneity in prevalence rates across studies. Studies have identified high rates of mental disorders in refugees, but most used self-report measures of psychiatric symptoms, unlike the screening program for the migration to the United States.

TABLE 11.4 Mental class status for refugees and immigrants from Iran, Iraq, Afghanistan and Syria

Country	Refugees			Immigrants			Total migrants		
	Mental class A&B (n)	Total (n)	Mental class A&B (%)	Mental class A&B (n)	Total (n)	Mental class A&B (%)	Mental class A&B (n)	Total (n)	Mental class A&B (%)
Iraq	645	10,037	5.1	110	2,811	2.1	755	12,848	4.1
Iran	392	3,790	9.1	1,617	21,161	6.1	2,009	24,951	7.1
Syria	544	6,241	7.1	21	752	1.1	561	6,993	7.1
Afghanistan	961	4,156	22.1	50	858	4.1	1,011	5,014	19.1
Overall	**2,542**	**24,224**	**9.1**	**1,798**	**25,582**	**6.1**	**4,336**	**49,806**	**7.1**

According to the International Rescue Committee (IRC), Iraqi refugees arrive in the United States with more emotional and mental health issues than many other refugee groups, and the IRC has documented a high prevalence of depression, anxiety and PTSD among recently arrived Iraqis. A 2009 study estimated the lifetime prevalence of any mental disorder at 18.8% for Iraqi adults. Anxiety disorders were the most common (13.8%) class of disorders in the cohort studied, and major depressive disorder was the most common (7.2%) single disorder. The numbers are considerable when considering that many migrants get health services from the GPs/FDs. The difference in screening periods may be an influencing factor. There are known factors such as an acculturation difficulty after arrival to the destination, which may trigger any underlying PTSD and depressive disorder. We screen prior to US migration, and the IRC numbers show those after migration has been completed, settling in the United States.

Although comparisons cannot be accurately made, one may see that the numbers are high in both the United States and Türkiye. Those living in the United States might be affected by many other factors, such as wrong expectations and reality, coping with status change, adjustment problems and acculturation difficulty.

SCREENING MIGRANTS AND REFUGEES IN TÜRKIYE

Our screening population is around 50,000, larger than many other studies on migrant mental health. We do not have the qualitative data here, nor can we include the distribution of diagnoses, but as violence has declined between 2005 and 2011, those Iraqi refugees living in Türkiye for a while probably have mental conditions other than PTSD. As that was a relatively quiet period, mental conditions may be similar to those immigrants. When the country was stable, the prevalence among immigrants was lower than that found in refugees.

Immigrant and refugee groups of the same nationality differ in prevalence for all nationalities. Syrian refugees who are escaping from a still partially active war may have more PTSD. We expect to see more numbers from Syria and other neighbours in coming years. Among 7,000 Syrians, 7.1% of mental cases are lower than expected, although considerably high. Also the number of Syrians who immigrate to the United States may increase as time passes. More than 200,000 Syrian migrants are Turkish citizens now. Some were born here, and some applied for passports and settled here, making a gross change in the demography of certain cities and regions. They brought their own culture; hence, the migrants expect the GPs/FDs to understand their culture and social structure while providing medical care.

The information provided here is intended to help resettlement agencies, GPs/FDs, other clinicians and health care providers understand the mental health issue of greatest concern pertaining to resettling refugee populations. This is based on our daily clinical experience and our expertise, and might be helpful to other colleagues with refugees in their daily practice.

MANIFESTATION OF MENTAL HEALTH ISSUES

We often see depression and anxiety together when screening refugees. Basically, refugees are already under intense stress; they are usually worried about many aspects of their lives, and usually they have marked anxiety, which a GP/FD may easily notice. What is interesting here is the refugees are all aware of this, and they relate/link and normalise this condition within their current status. However, they may not be aware that they are depressed. This is something really important for a GP/FD to know.

Refugees usually do not come with a current/acute psychiatric complaint. They often do not express their psychiatric complaints themselves, but these emerge when specific questions are asked. Routine psychiatric examination and initial questions used for depression, such as symptoms of sleep disorder and decreased interest may be asked, but a GP/FD shall keep in mind that these 'diagnostic questions lose their meaning' for this group, unlike other patients who seek help from a GP/FD. Kidnapping, abuse, violence and rape may have been normalised to the extent that they can be asked about in a routine question list, and especially domestic violence.

Every refugee entering the medical examination room is evaluated not only in terms of physical findings but also in terms of perception, orientation and mood. In addition, related core questions are asked regarding depression, anxiety and PTSD, according to the DSM-V. We ask these as family physicians/general practitioners in the migrant health screening practice. Validated tools and scales for primary care screening are applied with the help of an interpreter to communicate in the person's native language and not miss anything, especially the presence of impaired functionality, harmful behaviour history or harmful behaviour risk or the presence of any suicidal thoughts at any time. All are asked with clear sentences. Depending on our personal experience as experts in refugee screening, events such as rape, torture and suicide that are asked about in a clear and ordinary way makes the person being examined more comfortable and facilitates giving clear and real answers to the questions.

We screen, detect and manage each case after diagnosis, until the departure with a pre-flight evaluation, and also help with arrangements after arriving with filling in and submitting special medical condition forms to let the resettlement agencies in the United States know about the condition, how to follow up and what is needed after arrival. In cases where a harmful behaviour risk is high or cannot be classified according to the DSM-V and CDC TIs, refugees are re-evaluated by a psychiatrist in our clinic face-to-face (or rarely online in conditions like the recent pandemic). In addition, as they are usually living in satellite cities where they are settled by the Turkish government, as they are not officially living in Istanbul or in Ankara where we screen, we prepare and provide them with a detailed referral letter.

Türkiye's universal health system provides coverage of all health expenses for refugees – they can be treated in their cities the same as Turkish citizens. That is why they are referred to a psychiatric specialist in their own settlement city for treatment/follow-up if needed, in addition to regular follow-ups in our clinic by our own panel psychiatrist. We can call them back for a follow-up appointment the following month if necessary. They are paid by a resettlement agency for their travels, accommodation and daily expenses for this medical follow-up trip. Not only while they are living here in Türkiye as guests, we also indicate the necessity of follow-up for the resettlement process in the United States after arrival.

There are also cases where we refer patients with substance use for treatment to the Alcohol and Substance Treatment Center, an authorised governmental institution specialising in substance use disorders and management of diagnosed patients. This service is also free of charge for refugees.

HEALTH LITERACY

Although they have a similar rate of psychiatric disease burden to the society they live in, refugees do not have the same chance to access health services if no one guides them in the city/country where they are settled temporarily. They mostly do not have knowledge about where and how to access health services or how to reach psychiatry clinical services. On the other hand, especially in terms of psychiatric needs, they do not even think about seeking help regarding their housing, heating, food and work needs. They have accepted their current status of mind as a natural consequence of being a refugee. They show no effort or any search to get out of that situation. That is why screening, detecting and managing cases is of utmost importance to help such vulnerable people and also considering its importance for public health.

IMPROVEMENTS ARE NEEDED

Work is needed on specific tools for screening. Scales should be revised and validated for the refugee group. For example, asking questions such as 'Do you have sleep problems lately?' or 'Do you ever not enjoy things that used to make you happy?' to a woman who lost her husband in war, has one missing child, is unemployed, is homeless and has been living in a foreign country for five or six years where she does not speak the language is meaningless! Please feel empathy and then re-think the guidelines.

Suspicion/diagnosis of any psychiatric disease, aiming for a correct referral and finally classification of the applicant for migration are said to be the main role of a PP. But this is no different from primary health care (PHC) in terms of holistic health approach and community mental health. All PHC physicians, not just PPs, should apply these same principles. FDs/GPs should consider every patient who enters the examination room from a biopsychosocial well-being perspective, and especially migrant/refugee groups who have language barriers, cultural barriers, suppressed sexual identities in some cases and live far from their family/country and social support.

Every headache, angina and tachycardia should be questioned in terms of 'depression/anxiety/somatic' problems. Undiagnosed or untreated depression/anxiety can become treatment-resistant, leading to functional impairment, and may even result in suicide. These issues can become part of collective memory and be passed onto future generations. Suicidal thoughts, which are often suppressed for 'religious' reasons in the current generation, may emerge in the next generation.

Overall, migrant mental disorder prevalence for the eight-year period from 2014 to 2022 is 7.1%. There is a significant difference between the refugee and immigrant 'mental health disorders' overall prevalence (9.1% vs 6.1%). What does that mean? As primary care physicians, GPs/FDs, you need to be careful with these vulnerable people in primary care, as they will be searching for help.

REFERENCES

1. United Nations High Commissioner for Refugees. 2022. Available from: https://www.unhcr.org/data.html.
2. United Nations High Commissioner for Refugees. 2013 UNHCR country operations profile - Iraq. Available from: https://data.unhcr.org/en/country/irq.
3. Charlson F, van Ommeren M, Flaxman A et al (2019) New WHO prevalence estimates of mental disorders in conflict settings: a systematic review and meta-analysis. Lancet. doi: 10.1016/s0140-6736(19)30934-1

11.3 MENTAL HEALTH DISORDERS, ANXIETY AND DEPRESSION IN UKRAINIANS ASSOCIATED WITH WAR AND MIGRATION

Victoria Tkachenko

Mental health disorders are highly prevalent in all countries throughout the world. Every eighth person in the world lives with a mental disorder. The prevalence of different mental disorders (10–15%) varies with country, sex and age, but anxiety and depressive disorders are the most common.[1]

In Ukraine in 2015 the prevalence of depressive disorders was 6.3%, and anxiety disorders 3.2%, which was the highest in the WHO European region.[2] This was the result of additional triggers and risk factors such as military conflict in the eastern part of Ukraine with the displacement of people and an unstable political and economic situation.

A few years later, the WHO STEPs survey in 2019 showed that every eighth adult (12.4%) in Ukraine had reported symptoms consistent with a clinical diagnosis of depression. However, only every fourth person with probable depression (3% of the total population) had been told by a doctor or health care professional about it. Only 0.4% of the population had undergone treatment, either with antidepressant medication or psychological therapy – equivalent to a treatment coverage rate of only 3.2% of probable cases of depression.[3]

In 2020 the new global environmental trigger was added – the crisis caused by the COVID-19 pandemic. The measures imposed by governments such as isolation, quarantine, restrictions and social and economic instability led to a massive increase of 25% in terms of the prevalence of anxiety and depression globally, according to the WHO World Mental Health report.[1]

The full-scale war of Russia against Ukraine since 24 February 2022 became a new powerful psycho-traumatic event that affected people in Ukraine and all over the world. In addition, the process of informatisation, when everything happens almost live, with people watching online, including seeing bombings and deaths, has been an additional worsening factor. The impact of the war on mental health is likely to remain its most devastating and lasting legacy, mostly for Ukrainians.

The Ministry of Health of Ukraine reported that about 15 million citizens need professional psychological help and 3–4 million need psychotropic medications. The Gradus research showed that about 71% of Ukrainians have recently felt stress or strong nervousness, 50% feel anxiety and tension and 20–30% of people may develop PTSD.[4] At the same time, 49% of Ukrainian respondents believe that psychological help is only for mentally ill people, and more than 80% have never consulted a psychologist in their life. Only 2% of respondents have consulted a health practitioner – psychologist, psychotherapist, family doctor or therapist – about this. Additionally, the Ministry of Health of Ukraine predicts an increase in the number of drug, alcohol and other addictions in 5–7 years, with a huge increase in noncommunicable diseases at 10–15 years younger age than before the war.[4]

Mental disorders are a normal response to an abnormal situation; however, if they are not addressed in time, they can cause irreversible effects on public health. The anxiety, panic, mild or severe depression, insomnia and other stress-related disorders during the war are caused by such stressful situations as bombing, air raid warnings at day and night, hiding in basements from shelling, being in shelters or cellars (underground, cold, dark, closed places) for a long time, problems with delivery of food and medicines, trying to feed families after losing a job, problems with electricity and connection, facing power outages, leaving homes in search of safety and experiencing repeated displacements, destruction of homes, being separated from loved ones or being a refugee abroad without knowing the language.

While the greatest needs are recorded in the areas most affected by the war, people in relatively safe parts of Ukraine are also experiencing stress, and the lives of those who have gone abroad are clouded by the guilt of having left their home country during these critical times. The recent general population survey of the International Organization for Migration showed that every fourth Ukrainian (23%) needs mental health and psychosocial support among internally displaced people, as well as refugees.[5,6]

War, armed conflict and other man-made or natural disasters cause profound distress and can ignite or inflame existing mental health conditions. The WHO emphasises that among people who have experienced war or other conflict, most people will recover without help; however, one in five (22%) will have a mental health condition such as depression, anxiety or PTSD in the next 10 years, and one in ten will have a severe condition such as psychosis, bipolar disorder or schizophrenia.[7]

In order to provide high-quality and effective psychological assistance to affected Ukrainians, it is necessary to understand how exactly Ukrainians react to the war and the stress factors associated with it.

PORTRAIT OF UKRANIAN CLIENTS

The Institute of Social and Political Psychology of Ukraine conducted an online survey of the population in and outside of Ukraine. Forty percent of respondents experienced threats to their own lives and/or were direct witnesses of such threats in connection with being in a combat zone and/or under shelling. More than 41% of citizens have relatives or loved ones who were, or who are in the war zone, including 16% who have lost someone close to them; 6% of respondents were under occupation, were directly threatened with violence or witnessed such threats. Every twentieth interviewee (5%) experienced repeated and hence cumulative traumatisation – experiencing or witnessing numerous traumatic events such as shelling, threats to the lives of loved ones, occupation or captivity. Only 9% of citizens had experienced no traumatic event during the period of full-scale war. More than 90% of respondents had manifestations of at least one of the symptoms of PTSD, and 57% are at risk of developing PTSD.[8]

Those who applied for crisis counselling, as noted by the National Psychological Association of Ukraine, were mostly young women (90%) and far fewer men (10%); 84% sought crisis counselling after a specific traumatic event – the need to leave home (59%), death or threat to the life of a loved one (36%), threat to one's own life or lack of contact with loved ones (34%).

Emotional symptoms were much more pronounced than physical and cognitive symptoms. The most frequent emotional symptoms were constant tension and inability to relax (52%), anxiety (38%), fear (37%), guilt, survivor's syndrome (36%), emotional instability (34%), depressive states (26%), helplessness and despair (29%), apathy (14%), emotional freezing, poorly controlled aggression and panic attacks. Among the physical symptoms, the most frequent were sleep problems (45%), physical exhaustion and severe fatigue (34%), breathing problems, feeling of suffocation (30%), chest pain, palpitations (20%) and tremors (16%). Cognitive symptoms were overthinking (40%), problems with concentration (30%), inhibition of thinking and speech (24%), deterioration of memory and loss of events (9%).[9]

Those who remained in Ukraine experience more stress in terms of physical exhaustion, powerlessness, apathy and inability to decide whether to leave or stay. Among those who have gone abroad, issues include feelings of guilt, survivor's syndrome, concern for loved ones who remained in Ukraine, adaptation problems and the difficulty of deciding whether to stay or return home. Guilt for not fighting and loss of support are typical for men.[9]

Among the defence mechanisms, the displacement of the traumatic experience and suppression of emotions, devaluation, denial and projection were the most common. Among the coping strategies, seeking social support (61%), self-control strategies (37%) and acceptance of responsibility (38%) were frequent.[9]

However, a rapid situational analysis revealed that the feeling of connectedness with people, a sense of national identity and pride, selflessness and supporting others, religion and humour and laughter have contributed to the collective resilience of Ukrainians.[6,11]

The level of emotional solidarity with host communities as an indicator of the impact on psychological well-being as a result of internal migration is higher than average. At the same time, citizens are inclined to a passive or declarative type of solidarity – the presence of a positive attitude towards the host communities with a relatively low readiness to effectively integrate into them.[8]

About 70% respondents did not feel the need to seek psychological help, only 3% of respondents received such help and another 23% would like to.[8]

PRIMARY CARE MENTAL HEALTH SERVICES IN UKRAINE

Despite the high prevalence of mental disorders, the treatment gap remains large and is mainly attributed to legacy of the Semashko-style structure of the Ukrainian health care system. Mental health reform since 2017 is an integral component of the overall health care system transformation in Ukraine. The International Classification of Primary Care (ICPC-2) is implemented for primary care doctors who are allowed to register common mental health conditions (P01-P99), including such diagnoses as anxiety disorder (P74) and depressive disorder (P76). As for psychotherapeutists, they use International Classification of Diseases (ICD-10) classification and the spectrum of diagnoses F3 and F4.

State plans to improve mental health care until 2030 include the integration of mental health care in primary health care, provision of services through multidisciplinary teams and developing a system of psychological and social assistance at the community level.[10,11] Ukrainian family doctors started to be trained according to the WHO Mental Health Gap Action Programme (mhGAP),[12] which aims at scaling up services for mental, neurological and substance use and to improve access. In addition to health workers, social workers, police officers, volunteers and teachers will also be trained to provide basic services and support to patients with mental health conditions and disorders.[10,11]

Government-led efforts aimed at the long-term impact on mental health, including the National Programme on Mental Health and Psychosocial Support, were launched under the leadership of the first lady of Ukraine, Olena Zelenska, in 2022.[6]

International and national organisations are working on implementation of the operational roadmap titled 'Ukrainian Prioritized Multisectoral Mental Health and Psychosocial Support Actions During and After the War: Operational Roadmap'[13] that sets out priority actions in different sectors – including health, social work and education. It also supports the development of the mental health system in line with the best global practices.

SUMMARY

This chapter covers mental health disorders associated with Russian-Ukrainian war and migration, its features, concomitant symptoms and portraits of internal displaced Ukrainians and refugees and the results of studies in mental health as well as the description of the Ukrainian mental health care system, strategy and psychosocial supportive actions during and after the war.

REFERENCES

1. World Health Organization. World Mental Health Report: Transforming Mental Health for All. Geneva: World Health Organization. 2022. Licence: CC BY-NC-SA 3.0 IGO. https://www.who.int/publications/i/item/9789240049338 (accessed Dec 30, 2022).
2. World Health Organization. Depression and Other Common Mental Disorders: Global Health Estimates. Geneva: World Health Organization. 2017. Licence: CC BY-NC-SA 3.0 IGO. Available from: https://apps.who.int/iris/handle/10665/254610 (accessed Dec 30, 2022).

3. World Health Organization. Regional Office for Europe. STEPS: Prevalence of Noncommunicable Disease Risk Factors in Ukraine 2019. Copenhagen: WHO Regional Office for Europe. 2020. Licence: CC BY-NC-SA 3.0 IGO. Available from: https://apps. who.int/iris/handle/10665/336642 (accessed Dec 30, 2022).

4. Gradus Research. State of Ukrainians 'Mental Health'. Their Attitude Towards Psychological Help During the War. Gradus Research Plus. 2022. Available from: https://gradus.app/documents/313/Gradus_Research___Mental_Health_Report_ ENG.pdf (accessed Dec 30, 2022).

5. International Organization for Migration. Ukraine — Internal Displacement Report — General Population Survey Round 11 (25 November - 5 December 2022). International Organization for Migration (IOM), Ukraine Returns Report, December, 2022. Available from: https://displacement.iom.int/sites/g/files/tmzbdl1461/files/reports/ IOM_Gen%20Pop%20Report_R11_IDP_ENG_0.pdf (accessed Dec 30, 2022).

6. Anh N. How War and Displacement Affect Mental Health of People in Ukraine and Why We Should Address This. Available from: https://ukraine.iom.int/blogs/how-war-and-displacement-affect-mental-health-people-ukraine-and-why-we-should-address (accessed Dec 30, 2022).

7. Charlson F, van Ommeren M, Flaxman A, Cornett J, Whiteford H, Saxena S. New WHO prevalence estimates of mental disorders in conflict settings: a systematic review and meta-analysis. Lancet. 2019 Jul 20;394(10194):240–48. doi: 10.1016/S0140-6736(19)30934-1. Epub 2019 Jun 12.

8. Press release – Study of the psychological state of the population in conditions of full-scale war. Available from: https://ispp.org.ua/2022/09/13/doslidzhennya-psixologichnogo-stanu-naselennya-v-umovax-povnomasshtabnoii-vijni/ (accessed Dec 30, 2022).

9. Ovchar O, Bolman S. Results of the Research 'Mental State of Pre-War-Time Anti-Russia Ukrainians'. NPAU. 2022. https://drive.google.com/file/d/1hsNwEdq32p4a5au a24NIQpd6ltiyY8mW/view?fbclid=IwAR0OLmHOzLs84pJyFSyXZ_75vtAml3o9hUq EXzG-_9OSmwHArotTrpBfJeU (accessed Dec 30, 2022).

10. Inka W, Khan O, Kondakova N, Poole LA, Cohen JT. Mental health in transition: assessment and guidance for strengthening integration of mental health into primary health care and community-based service platforms in Ukraine: Психічне здоров'я на перехідному етапі: оцінка та керівництво для посилення інтеграції психічного здоров'я (Ukrainian). Global Mental Health Initiative Washington, D.C.: World Bank Group. 2018. Available from: http://documents.worldbank.org/curated/ en/747231517553325438/Психічне-здоровя-на-перехідному-етапі-оцінка-та-керівництво-для-посилення-інтеграції-психічного-здоровя (accessed Dec 30, 2022).

11. World Health Organization. Mental Health & Psychosocial Support Rapid Situational Analysis Ukraine—Kyiv, Odessa & Lviv. April 2022. World Health Organization. 2022. https://www.humanitarianresponse.info/sites/www.humanitarianresponse.info/files/ documents/files/imc_2022_ukraine_mhpss_rapid_situational_analysis.pdf (accessed Dec 30, 2022).

12. World Health Organization. mhGAP Intervention Guide for Mental, Neurological and Substance Use Disorders in Non-Specialized Health Settings: Mental Health Gap Action Programme (mhGAP), Version 2.0. World Health Organization; 2016. https:// apps.who.int/iris/handle/10665/250239 (accessed Dec 30, 2022).

13. World Health Organization. Ukrainian Prioritized Multisectoral Mental Health and Psychosocial Support Actions During and After the War: Operational Roadmap. Open Document (5 December 2022). World Health Organization. 2022. https://www. humanitarianresponse.info/sites/www.humanitarianresponse.info/files/documents/ files/mhpss_framework_ukraine_eng_ok_v18.pdf (accessed Dec 30, 2022).

CHAPTER 12

Interventions for treating depression and anxiety in primary care

DOI: 10.1201/9781003391531-12

12.1 'WATCHFUL WAITING' – A POWERFUL APPROACH

Anna Stavdal and Susan Senstad

> Primary care doctors have both a generalist's education, including in psychiatry, and a unique possibility to learn about the life challenges their patients face. Consequently, they should be patients' first point of contact when psychological dysfunctions manifest.
>
> *Lars Lien, Board Chairman*
> *Norwegian Psychiatric Association*[1]

Many of us assume, perhaps without realising it, that our aim as medical doctors is to diagnose and cure disease. Then, when no diagnosis fits and no cure exists, we conclude that we have failed. Our primary obligation, regardless of our specialty, is actually far broader: To identify and mitigate health issues to the maximum extent that our most current 'best practice' permits. From that perspective, it becomes essential first to distinguish disease from non-disease and then to choose our approach accordingly. Every family doctor does that every single day.

Making such distinctions becomes increasingly difficult, however, as psychological jargon seeps into our everyday speech. Those admitting that they 'feel down' are quickly characterised as 'depressed', as if they met the criteria of that mental illness term. Meantime, people who pathologically lack access to appropriate emotional responses to losses and crises are likely to be labelled as being 'just fine'.

The more that daily life is medicalised, the less capable people become of recognising actual pathology when they see it and leaving open spaces for normality. Primary care providers with 'watchful waiting' in their repertoire are well-positioned to put the brakes on this trend by sorting symptoms of a mental illness from normal reactions to situational crises.

WHAT IS 'WATCHFUL WAITING'?

'Watchful waiting' can be a Family Doctor's 'best practice' with patients experiencing mental health concerns, including those at most points along the continuum of what we refer to as 'depression'. It's easier to describe its use, however, with a straightforward, somatic example as follows:

Let's say that a patient consults a family doctor because of an earache. We doctors know that otalgia might be an early sign of a cranial tumour. Because it is far more likely to indicate otitis, however, we explain to the patient that it makes sense to give the situation time to resolve itself, with or without some treatment. We explain that we hope to avoid putting them through unnecessary testing, but, if their pain persists, we will make sure that the right diagnostic examinations are carried out. Meantime, we'll wait watchfully, together.

SOME CLINICIAN/PATIENT BENEFITS OF 'WATCHFUL WAITING'

Our 'watchful waiting' strengthens our capacity to resist the pressure – and the temptation – to rush to diagnose, to medicate, to refer. Instead, we can allow a mutual recognition of a suitable diagnosis to emerge, as well as clarity about which, if any, medications might prove useful. Then, if we do decide to refer the patient to another level of care, the hand-over process can model for patients how to navigate the health care system on their own behalf, carefully and well. By contrast, any uncritical pursuit of 'early detection' seems both disrespectful and risky.

Our 'watchful waiting' treatment plan timeframe is determined by the patient's own development and experience of symptoms. A treatment that has been designed in cooperation with, and tailored to, one specific person at that unique moment in life tends to provoke far fewer compliance issues. Once people are cast by the medical model into the role of 'patient', their sense of identity may be defined and delimited by their diagnosis; it's as if that entire person were now nothing more than 'mentally ill'. The relational process of 'watchful waiting', however, may soothe the stinging shame that so often accompanies diagnoses, encouraging patients both to view and experience themselves as whole human beings.

Sending the implicit message, 'I will follow you, as your witness and companion', we help prepare our patients to recognise and adapt to the inevitable crises of life. As we ask them to join us in watching for what might trigger their symptoms, worsen, or relieve them, they learn to attend more acutely to the nuances of their lived body. As we watch and wait together, we allow the logic embedded in patients' strategies for tackling existential struggles to be revealed; we can then take the time we need to consider alternatives that might serve them better.

Allowing time to pass in a context of supportive awareness allows patients to define time as a resource. Their capacity for patience increases as it becomes associated more with self-respect and relational respect than, for example, traumatic neglect. The patient/doctor relationship, that core agent of healing, is likely to deepen. Thus, the 'watchful waiting' process as a whole may function as a subtle form of 'corrective experience over time', strengthening the very foundations of patients' mental health.

CHALLENGES

Of course, 'watchful waiting' might cost us money. We may be diagnosing less while working in a system that pays more for work done with severe diagnoses. We may prescribe fewer psychopharmaceuticals in a place where big pharma offers tempting 'incentives'.

We may not even get as many opportunities for using 'watchful waiting' with mental health distress as with more overtly somatic issues. For one thing, primary care patients may resist asking us for help, given the intractable stigma tied to mental illness. And we may be keeping them away. The symptoms of mental health issues don't lend themselves easily to objective assessment; we may worry that the in-depth communication needed to reveal the nature and severity of the problem might consume too much of our already overbooked time. By inadvertently communicating such resistance, we may trigger patients' fears of being unable to 'prove' there is something wrong. They may respond to our 'watchful waiting' idea as if we were rejecting them, refusing to treat them. They may protest that we're 'not doing anything' for them.

They may indeed be right – if we have confused 'watchful waiting' with 'doing nothing for a while'. Using 'watchful waiting' responsibly requires mental health proficiencies that not many schools teach. We need to become adept at reading between life's lines, with informed compassion, experiential insight, and problem-solving knowledge. We must be prepared to set appropriate boundaries while still maintaining an authentic emotional presence. Trying to fake it may do damage, leaving patients with their issues unaddressed and their negative expectations confirmed.

In short, we primary care physicians – in fact, all mental health workers including psychiatrists – would surely benefit from reviving the psychoanalytic practice of undergoing 'a control analysis'. Socrates revealed the secret to practicing high-quality 'watchful waiting': 'Know thyself'.

REFERENCE

1. Lien L. Folkeopplysningen's episode "Psych" is misleading. Aftenposten, Norway. Oct 4, 2022 [AS translation]. Available from: https://www.aftenposten.no/meninger/kronikk/i/l3V9wL/folkeopplysningens-episode-psyk-er-misvisende

12.2 PSYCHOTHERAPEUTIC INTERVENTIONS FOR DEPRESSION AND ANXIETY IN PRIMARY CARE

Vinicius Jobim Fischer, Raquel Gómez Bravo and Alice Einloft Brunnet

INTRODUCTION

As previously outlined in this book, depression and anxiety disorders are two of the most common mental disorders worldwide with a projected lifetime risk of up to 36% for any anxiety disorder and up to 31% for any mood disorder.[1] Epidemiological studies estimated a 12-month prevalence for depression of up to 7% for men and 11% for women and between 7% and 9% for men and 15% to 18% for women for anxiety disorders.[2-4] Such conditions implicate a wide range of impairments, impacting the society and the economy due to the deterioration of the performance at school, productivity at work and social and family relationships which, in summary, hampers one's capacity to take part in the community.[5]

According to the 11th revision of the International Classification of Diseases (ICD-11), depression and anxiety are grouped under the mental, behavioural and neurodevelopmental disorders.[6] Depressive disorders are mood disorders characterised by depressive mood (e.g., sadness, irritability, emptiness) or loss of pleasure accompanied by other cognitive, behavioural or neurovegetative symptoms which significantly affect one's functionality with significant distress or impairment in personal, family, social, educational and occupational spheres. Other common symptoms are decreased energy levels, disruptions in sleep or eating, difficulties in concentration and decision making, and withdrawal from social activities. The consequences of depression can be recurrent or long-lasting and can dramatically affect a person's ability to function and live a rewarding life. Moreover, depression is the leading cause of disability around the world and contributes greatly to the general global burden of disease.[5,7]

If someone has previously experienced a manic, mixed or hypomanic episode, a depressive disorder diagnosis should not be given, and a bipolar disorder should be considered. Furthermore, the clinical manifestation should not be accounted for by another medical condition, nor due to the effects of a substance or medication (e.g., alcohol, benzodiazepine) on the central nervous system, including withdrawal effects (e.g., from cocaine).

Anxiety and fear-related disorders are defined by excessive fear and anxiety and related behavioural disturbances, with manifestations which are severe enough to result in significant distress or significant impairment in personal, family, social, educational, occupational or other important areas of functioning. Both fear and anxiety are closely related phenomena; the first indicates a reaction to a perceived imminent threat in the present, whereas the second is more future-oriented, referring to a perceived anticipated threat (ICD-11).

In this context, pivotal differentiating features of anxiety and fear-related disorders are disorder-specific foci of apprehension; in other words, there is a stimulus or situation that triggers the fear or anxiety. Clinical presentation commonly includes specific associated cognitions which can assist in the diagnosis differentiation among the disorders by clarifying the focus of apprehension. This focus may be very specific (such as in specific phobias) or relate to a broader sort of situation (as in generalised anxiety disorder) (ICD-11). There are seven anxiety and fear-related disorder diagnoses: Generalised anxiety disorder, panic disorder, agoraphobia, specific phobia, social anxiety disorder, separation anxiety disorder, selective mutism and other specified anxiety or fear-related disorders. The causes of depression and anxiety disorders encompass a complex interaction between biological, social and psychological factors. To name a few, childhood adversity, loss and unemployment may contribute to or generate the development of depression.

There are psychological and pharmacological treatments for depression and anxiety. However especially in low- and middle-income countries (LMICs), treatment and support services for mental disorders are often underdeveloped or absent. It is estimated that in LMICs more than 75% of people suffering from mental disorders do not receive treatment.[5] In response to the dramatic impact of depression and anxiety on the global burden of disease and disability, the World Health Organization (WHO) has developed a series of proposals. One of them is the *Mental Health Gap Action Programme (mhGAP)*, a mental health intervention guide for the identification and treatment and follow-up of mental, neurological and substance use disorders in non-specialised health settings. This programme, initially developed in 2008 and in constant evolution, provides guidance for clinical decision-making. It offers some guidance regarding transversal abilities needed to address mental health concerns, such as effective communication skills. Six tips are mentioned (Figure 12.1): (1) Create an environment that facilitates open communication; (2) involve the person; (3) start by listening; (4) be friendly, respectful and non-judgmental at all times; (5) use good verbal communication skills; and (6) respond with sensitivity when people disclose difficult experiences such as sexual assault, violence or self-harm.

Another initiative is the programme management plus (PM+) intervention, a brief psychological intervention for adults which targets the offer of individual psychological help for adults impaired by distress in communities exposed to adversity. The PM+ intervention made changes to highly specialised training in cognitive behavioural therapy (CBT) in order to be simpler and scalable, requesting fewer trained human resources (also called 'low-intensity psychological interventions'). In other words, community health workers with or without previous training in mental health care are able to provide it effectively as long as they are trained and supervised.[8] The

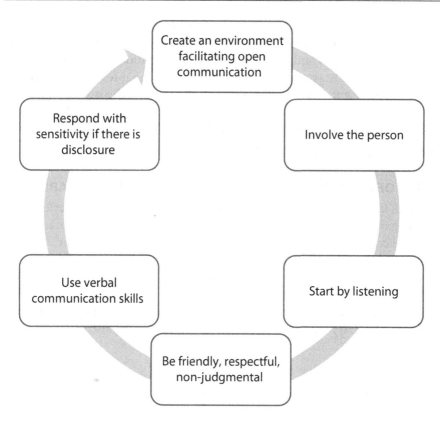

FIGURE 12.1 Transversal abilities to address mental health concerns.

intervention combines problem management (problem-solving therapy or problem-solving counselling) and behavioural strategies.

DEPRESSION AND ANXIETY IN PRIMARY CARE

The high prevalence of these mental health disorders stresses the importance of addressing them at the primary care level, offering mental health services and different treatment options to the population. Delivery of treatment in primary care settings may be more effective in overcoming disparities in access and use, as this may overcome barriers to care and have less accompanying stigma than accessing a specialty mental health care setting.[9]

Comprehensive mental health care in the primary-level settings should foster communication with the patient and caregivers, stress reduction, social support strengthening and daily activities promotion. In other words, the primary health care provider's aim is to facilitate cognitive, behavioural or emotional adjustments, increasing the patients' symptoms remission odds, or, in the worst scenarios, enabling them to deal better with their symptom manifestations.

Depression and anxiety share the same underlying core structure, symptoms and maintaining factors.[10,11] Furthermore, they tend to respond similarly to psychological and pharmacological interventions.[12] In primary care, interventions such as the ones discussed in this chapter are particularly valuable because they are transdiagnostic in nature, being useful even if the clinician has difficulty establishing a differential diagnosis.[13] Indeed, rather than giving patients a diagnostic label, it may be better for the clinician to talk about helping to address their distress.

TYPES OF PSYCHOSOCIAL INTERVENTIONS IN PRIMARY CARE

A health intervention can be defined as "any action destined to interfere with and stop or modify a process, as in treatment undertaken to halt, manage, or alter the course of the pathological process of a disease or disorder".[14] When there is a lack of highly specialised trained professionals, attention must be given to the selection of the intervention, the setting availability and the willingness and ability of the patient to proceed with the treatment.[15] There are a number of different techniques that can be taught and specific interventions applied in primary care aimed at reducing psychological distress.

Psychoeducation

Psychoeducation is an intervention aimed at giving individuals information about their condition, treatment options with respective duration, benefits of adherence and potential side effects.[16] This education intends to change their cognitions, beliefs, affect and behaviours and can be delivered in formal groups (psychoeducational groups) or as a routine part of initiating a treatment and follow-up plan.[17] For example, this might demystify a disorder to a patient and provide information about causes, symptoms and treatment options.

Relaxation training

Muscle- or breathing-relaxation techniques can aid in the treatment of emotional tension. For example, the rationale of relaxation exercises can be explained and patients taught how to practice relaxation and how to incorporate this into their routine.[18] Progressive muscle relaxation, also known as Jacobson relaxation, is a muscle relaxation technique which aims to relax the entire body by becoming aware of tensions in various muscle groups and then relaxing one muscle group at a time. In order to achieve the relaxation, the individual intentionally tenses specific muscles or muscle groups and then releases tension to achieve relaxation throughout the body.[19] Breathing relaxation is a technique which teaches patients slow diaphragmatic breathing through different methods, including therapist modelling and corrective feedback, particularly useful in the treatment of anxiety disorders and in the hyperventilation in panic disorder.

Mindfulness

An operational definition of mindfulness is "the awareness that emerges through paying attention on purpose, in the present moment, and nonjudgmentally to the unfolding of experience moment by moment".[20] Mindfulness refers to exercises of conscious effort to be attentive to the present moment in a non-judgmental way. The technique consists of an invitation to oneself to pay attention to one's senses in the 'here and now'. Such a strategy helps the patient to be in the present moment, avoiding the fearful worrying and/or anticipation of possible negative outcomes of future situations.

There are also a number of specific psychotherapies available to treat depression and anxiety in primary care. There is strong evidence that they are more effective than pharmacotherapy, although the effects are modest. Psychotherapy alone, or in combination with pharmacotherapy, has been shown to be more effective than pharmacotherapy alone both in getting depressed patients well and in keeping them well over time.[21]

Behavioural activation

Behavioural activation is aimed at increasing an individual's engagement in valued life activities through guided goal setting to bring about improvements in thoughts, mood and quality of life.[22] For example, this might involve inviting the person to engage in physical activity or in an activity that they have enjoyed in the past. It is based on the theory that when people become depressed, they tend to withdraw and become isolated, and engaging in these activities can improve their mood. Individuals may be asked to keep an activity schedule as part of the intervention.

Problem-solving therapy

Problem-solving therapy (PST) is a brief and focused psychological strategy which helps people learn skills for managing daily life problems, rather than focusing on directly modifying their thoughts and feelings. It provides patients with tools to identify and solve problems that arise from both big and small stressors in their lives. One problem-solving technique uses a stepwise approach: First identifying the real-life problem that needs to be solved and formulating it in a way that allows potential solutions to be generated; next to brainstorm possible solution options; thirdly discussing strategies to make decisions and overcome barriers; and lastly implementing a chosen solution and then checking whether it was effective in addressing the problem.

Interpersonal therapy

Interpersonal therapy (IPT) focuses on relieving symptoms of distress by improving interpersonal functioning. It looks at current problems and relationships, not backward at childhood or developmental issues. Therapists offer options to change problematic interpersonal behaviour patterns. It can be offered individually or in group settings. In the latter, participants have the opportunity to gain valuable insights while learning to relate to each other and then to apply those insights in their everyday lives outside of the group setting. It emphasises the curative influence of exploring the interactions of group members, including the analysis of group events, experiences and relationships. The therapist/facilitator can support the strengthening of the social support network. Patients with similar disorders can attend the same group to exchange the manner with which they deal with their condition and build up strategies to address the challenges they face.

Cognitive behavioural therapy

CBT is a form of psychotherapy that integrates theories of cognition and learning with treatment techniques. CBT assumes that cognitive, emotional and behavioural variables (what you think, feel and do) are functionally interrelated. Treatment is aimed at identifying and modifying maladaptive thought processes and problematic behaviours through cognitive restructuring and behavioural techniques to achieve a change in mood.[23] Cognitive restructuring is based on the identification of negative thought patterns or cognitive distortions – the health care professional helps the patient to identify them. Once patients are aware of them, they can learn how to reframe those thoughts in a less biased and more positive manner. For example, the depressed thought 'I blame myself for not being active/happy' can be reframed to 'blaming myself is unfair and makes dealing with my depression harder'.

Thought records or journalling involves inviting patients to keep track of their thoughts between sessions. In a follow-up session, alternative thoughts can be elicited and discussed. Alternatively, the health care provider can also suggest that the patient list new thoughts or new behaviours put into practice between sessions. For example, cognitive distortions such as 'I feel this way because I'm lazy' or 'I should blame myself for not being happy' can be identified. Patients can be helped to be self-aware when such thoughts appear and to respond to them.

COMPARABLE EFFECTIVENESS OF DIFFERENT PSYCHOTHERAPEUTIC INTERVENTIONS

Different psychological treatments have comparable effectiveness, and there are no clinically significant differences between them.[24] This includes behavioural activation, PST, IPT and brief forms of CBT, all interventions which can be used in primary care settings. The common core elements which contribute to their effectiveness have not yet been established.[25] These interventions can also have significant effects on secondary outcomes such as quality of life, social functioning, self-esteem and dysfunctional thinking.[26]

Delivery format

Psychotherapy can be delivered in many different formats: Face-to-face individually or in groups, over the telephone or as guided self-help delivered over the internet. There is little difference in effectiveness between these formats.[27] Internet (e-health) psychotherapies have a huge potential to reach large groups of patients in primary care and hence be cost-effective. A meta-analysis on the effectiveness and cost-effectiveness of e-health interventions for depression and anxiety in primary care found them to be moderately effective for depression when compared to waitlist and to have a small effect when compared to care as usual. However, this study highlighted the scarcity of evidence for the effectiveness of e-health interventions for anxiety in primary care.[28] While early research findings are promising, further work, including high-quality clinical trials, is needed for evidence that online interventions improve access to mental health treatment.[29,30]

CULTURAL AND CONTEXTUAL PERSPECTIVES IN THE PROVISION AND EVALUATION OF PSYCHOSOCIAL INTERVENTIONS IN PRIMARY CARE

Healthcare professionals in different countries are confronted with culturally diverse populations and frequently need to adapt their interventions to the context in which the patient lives. Addressing cultural and contextual issues during the entire health care process, from evaluation to intervention, is therefore essential to provide adequate care in mental health. In order to accomplish this goal, one essential asset for health care providers is cultural competence.

Cultural competence is an ongoing process, which can be continuously improved over time and can be defined as "the ability to work and communicate effectively and appropriately with people from culturally different backgrounds".[31] It is considered a multidimensional construct, which encompasses the healthcare professionals' cultural skills, cultural awareness and cultural knowledge.[31,32] Cultural skill is the ability to communicate and to interact with culturally different people; cultural awareness involves the awareness of the professional own's cultural features and values, and cultural knowledge is the continued acquisition of information about other cultures.[31,32] The number of studies testing the effects of cultural competence training on health care professionals' skills is increasing. Nonetheless, very few studies have verified the impact of the training both on health outcomes and on patient satisfaction/trust. More studies are still needed to develop evidence-based approaches in this field.[33]

Cultural competence is a clinical posture that has to be maintained throughout a patient's care provision. For this reason, culturally sensitive tools have been developed to assess cultural competence during all stages of care. Efforts have been made to improve the cultural sensibility of the recent versions of the international diagnoses manuals, the ICD-11 and *Diagnostic and Statistical Manual of Mental Disorders, Fifth Edition, Text Revision* (DSM-5-TR), which may help prevent inaccurate assessment in cross-cultural situation. This is a semi-structured assessment in four domains: (1) Cultural definition of a problem; (2) cultural perceptions of cause, context and support; (3) cultural factors affecting self-coping and past help seeking; and (4) cultural factors affecting current help seeking.[34] This interview may help assess some specific culture-related symptoms as well as how symptoms are interpreted by the patient and his or her community.

Studies have indeed shown variations among cultures regarding anxiety and depression symptom expression. For many cultural groups, the clinical presentation of anxiety may have a predominance of somatic complaints over cognitive symptoms. In addition, in some cultural contexts, symptoms of fear and anxiety may be reported primarily with reference to external forces or factors (for example, witchcraft, malign magic, sorcery or envy) and not as an internal experience or psychological state.[6] A similar pattern has been shown for depression: Cultures in which mental and physical health are viewed as interlinked tend to report more somatic than cognitive symptoms.[35]

Given that symptom expression and interpretation, including help-seeking behaviour, and other factors vary between cultures, it is essential to adapt an intervention protocol for patients' cultures and contexts. In a 2013 review, van Loon et al. evaluated culturally adapted guidelines for depression and anxiety in the United States.[36] Adaptations often included ethnic and language adaptation; incorporation of cultural values, beliefs and culturally specific symptoms; collaboration with culture brokers/mediators; adaptation of treatment time; and discussion about the therapeutic relationship. The culturally adapted protocols proved to be effective for US minority patients from different cultural backgrounds. A further meta-analysis described a moderate to large effect for culturally adapted interventions,[37] similar to those described by van Loon et al.[36] In most studies the protocols are adapted from 'western' to 'non-western' cultures, without taking into account the plurality of the latter.[37]

RECOMMENDATIONS FOR THE FUTURE

Depression and anxiety are two of the biggest mental health concerns. In addition to the lack of specialised trained professionals available, mental ill health and disorders still carry a series of barriers such as stigmas and taboos.

In addition to the societal prejudices towards such disorders, there is still a misconception that mental health care can only be provided by specialists.

From a clinical perspective, with this book, and particularly with this chapter, we hope to encourage primary care providers of different backgrounds and degrees of specialisation to provide care for depression and anxiety. From a research perspective, future research should examine whether varying levels of qualification among primary care CBT and other psychotherapy practitioners impacts on the effectiveness of CBT in this setting.[29] In order to provide effective and adequate treatment for depression and anxiety, it is essential that proper training is offered to the health care professionals who are in close contact with the patients. In consonance with the recommendations made by the WHO, training should be conducted by a mental health professional competent and experienced with psychological strategies used for such conditions. Essentially, trainings should encompass (1) information about depression and anxiety, (2) the rationale behind the application of each of the strategies, (3) strategies skills training, (4) role-playing of techniques (trainer demonstrations and trainee participation) and (5) helper self-care.[38]

Equally important is the offer of qualified supervision. Adequate supervision involves the space for the discussion about patients' progress, the exchange of difficulties experienced when applying the strategies with patients and the opportunity to practice skills and role-play how to manage difficult situations. Supervision can be delivered in different formats, including one-to-one, group or peer support group supervision.[38] Importantly, such activity can be done online with positive effects as well as face-to-face.[39] A minimum frequency and a limited number of participants per supervision session should be established (PM+ suggests two to three hours per week for group supervisions).[38]

CONCLUSIONS

This chapter aimed to present several low-intensity interventions for depression and anxiety that can be applied at the primary care level. Although two different diagnoses, the techniques presented here are transdiagnostic, meaning that they can be addressed to both conditions, as they tackle commonalities in the way patients often interpret and experience depression and anxiety. Our intention was to bring easily applicable strategies that can be applied in different cultural contexts. The cognitive and behavioural techniques described here are feasible to be implemented at the primary care level of attention. Such techniques can be learned and implemented by professionals without previous specialised training or formation. Specific training and supervision are enough in order to provide effectively the techniques mentioned. Although sometimes difficult to obtain, further education and supervision should always be sought.

Despite being effective, such techniques will not always be sufficient to induce remission of the symptoms or distress. Numbers needed to treat are often about four or five, meaning that only a minority of patients will benefit. It is pivotal to keep in mind that primary care is one level of care provision, but special attention must constantly be paid to patient progress and discussed with supervisors. In the cases in which improvement is deemed insufficient by the health provision team, several options should be considered, including continuation of the strategies used and follow-up with the patients or the referral of the patient to a (mental) health professional for assessment and further care.

REFERENCES

1. Kessler RC, Angermeyer M, Anthony JC, et al. Lifetime prevalence and age-of-onset distributions of mental disorders in the World Health Organization's world mental health survey initiative. World Psychiatry. 2007;6:168–76.
2. Ayuso-Mateos JL, Vazquez-Barquero JL, Dowrick C, et al. Depressive disorders in Europe: prevalence figures from the ODIN study. Br J Psychiatry. 2001;179:308–16.
3. Wittchen HU, Jacobi F. Size and burden of mental disorders in Europe—a critical review and appraisal of 27 studies. Eur Neuropsychopharmacol. 2005;15:357–76.
4. Kringlen E, Torgersen S, Cramer V. A Norwegian psychiatric epidemiological study. Am J Psychiatry. 2001;158:1091–8.
5. World Health Organization. Health Topics: Depression. 2022, November 24. Available from: https://www.who.int/health-topics/depression#tab=tab_1
6. World Health Organization. International statistical classification of diseases and related health problems. 11th ed. 2019. https://icd.who.int/
7. American Psychological Association. Dictionary of Psychology: Depression. 2022, August 8. Available from: https://dictionary.apa.org/depression
8. World Health Organization. Problem Management Plus (PM+): Individual Psychological Help for Adults Impaired by Distress in Communities Exposed to Adversity. (Generic field-trial version 1.1). Geneva: WHO. 2018.
9. Alegria M, Alvarez K, Ishikawa RZ, DiMarzio K, McPeck S. Removing obstacles to eliminating racial and ethnic disparities in behavioral health care. Health Aff. 2016;35:991–9. doi: 10.1377/hlthaff.2016.0029
10. Andrews G, Goldberg DP, Krueger RF, et al. Exploring the feasibility of a meta-structure for DSM-V and ICD-11: could it improve utility and validity? Psychol Med. 2009;39(12):1993–2000. doi: 10.1017/S0033291709990250
11. Harvey AG, Watkins E, Mansell W, Shafran R (Eds.). Cognitive behavioural processes across psychological disorders: a transdiagnostic approach to research and treatment. Oxford: Oxford University Press; 2004.
12. Hofmann SG, Asnaani A, Vonk IJ, Sawyer AT, Fang A. The Efficacy of cognitive behavioral therapy: a review of meta-analyses. Cognit Ther Res. 2012;36(5):427–40. doi: 10.1007/s10608-012-9476-1
13. Wittchen HU, Kessler RC, Beesdo K, Krause P, Höfler M, Hoyer J. Generalized anxiety and depression in primary care: prevalence, recognition, and management. J Clin Psychiatry. 2002;63(Suppl 8):24–34.
14. American Psychological Association. Dictionary of Psychology: Intervention. 2022, August 8. Available from: https://dictionary.apa.org/intervention
15. American Psychological Association. Dictionary of Psychology: Client-Education. 2022, August 8. Available from: https://dictionary.apa.org/client-education

16. World Health Organization. Mental health atlas 2014. World Health Organization; 2015. https://apps.who.int/iris/handle/10665/178879

17. American Psychological Association. Dictionary of Psychology: Interpersonal Group Psychotherapy. 2022, August 8. Available from: https://dictionary.apa.org/interpersonal-group-psychotherapy

18. American Psychological Association. Dictionary of Psychology: Breathing Retraining. 2022, August 8. Available from: https://dictionary.apa.org/breathing-retraining

19. American Psychological Association. Dictionary of Psychology: Progressive Relaxation. 2022, August 8. Available from: https://dictionary.apa.org/progressive-relaxation

20. Kabat-Zinn J. Mindfulness-based interventions in context: past, present, and future. Clin Psychol Sci Pract. 2003;10(2):144–56. doi: 10.1093/clipsy.bpg016

21. Furukawa TA, Shinohara K, Sahker E, Karyotaki E, Miguel C, Ciharova M, Bockting CLH, Breedvelt JF, Tajika A, Imai H, Ostinelli EG, Sakata M, Toyomoto R, Kishimoto S, Ito M, Furukawa Y, Cipriani A, Hollon SD, Cuijpers P. Initial treatment choices to achieve sustained response in major depression: a systematic review and network meta-analysis. World Psychiatry. 2021;20:387–96. doi: 10.1002/wps.20906

22. American Psychological Association. Dictionary of Psychology: Behavioral Activation. 2022, August 8. Available from: https://dictionary.apa.org/behavioral-activation

23. American Psychological Association. Dictionary of Psychology: Cognitive Behavior Therapy. 2022, August 8. Available from: https://dictionary.apa.org/cognitive-behavior-therapy

24. Cuijpers P, Gentili C. Psychological treatments are as effective as pharmacotherapies in the treatment of adult depression: a summary from randomized clinical trials and neuroscience evidence. Res Psychother. 2017;20(2):273. doi: 10.4081/ripppo.2017.273

25. Cuijpers P, Cristea IA, Karyotaki E, Reijnders M, Hollon SD. Component studies of psychological treatments of adult depression: a systematic review and meta-analysis. Psychother Res. 2019;29(1):15–29. doi: 10.1080/10503307.2017.1395922

26. Kolovos S, Kleiboer A, Cuijpers P. Effect of psychotherapy for depression on quality of life: meta-analysis. Br J Psychiatry. 2016;209(6):460–8.

27. Cuijpers P, Noma H, Karyotaki E, Cipriani A, Furukawa TA. Effectiveness and acceptability of cognitive behavior therapy delivery formats in adults with depression: a network meta-analysis. JAMA Psychiatry. 2019;76(7):700–07. doi: 10.1001/jamapsychiatry.2019.0268

28. Massoudi B, Holvast F, Bockting CLH, Burger H, Blanker MH. The effectiveness and cost-effectiveness of e-health interventions for depression and anxiety in primary care: a systematic review and meta-analysis. J Affect Disord. 2019;245:728–43. doi: 10.1016/j.jad.2018.11.050

29. Lehtimaki S, Martic J, Wahl B, Foster KT, Schwalbe N. Evidence on digital mental health interventions for adolescents and young people: systematic overview. JMIR Ment Health. 2021;8(4):e25847. doi: 10.2196/25847. PMID: 33913817; PMCID: PMC8120421.

30. Philippe TJ, Sikder N, Jackson A, et al. Digital health interventions for delivery of mental health care: systematic and comprehensive meta-review. JMIR Ment Health. 2022;9(5):e35159. Published 2022 May 12. doi:10.2196/35159

31. Alizadeh S, Chavan M. Cultural competence dimensions and outcomes: a systematic review of the literature. Health Soc Care Community. 2016;24(6):e117–e30. doi: 10.1111/hsc.12293

32. Kaihlanen AM, Hietapakka L, Heponiemi T. Increasing cultural awareness: qualitative study of nurses' perceptions about cultural competence training. BMC Nurs. 2019;18:38. Published 2019 Aug 22. doi: 10.1186/s12912-019-0363-x

33. Jongen C, McCalman J, Bainbridge R. Health workforce cultural competency interventions: a systematic scoping review. BMC Health Serv Res. 2018;18(1):232. Published 2018 Apr 2. doi: 10.1186/s12913-018-3001-5

34. American Psychiatric Association. Diagnostic and statistical manual of mental disorders. 5th ed. American Psychiatric Association; 2013.

35. Loveys K, Torrez J, Fine A, Moriarty G, Coppersmith G (2018). Cross-cultural differences in language markers of depression online. Proceedings of the 5th Workshop on Computational Linguistics and Clinical Psychology: From Keyboard to Clinic, CLPsych 2018 at the 2018 Conference of the North American Chapter of the Association for Computational Linguistics: Human Language Technologies, 78–87. doi: 10.18653/v1/w18-0608

36. van Loon A, van Schaik A, Dekker J, Beekman A. Bridging the gap for ethnic minority adult outpatients with depression and anxiety disorders by culturally adapted treatments. J Affect Disord. 2013;147(1–3):9–16. doi: 10.1016/j.jad.2012.12.014

37. Rathod S, Gega L, Degnan A, et al. The current status of culturally adapted mental health interventions: a practice-focused review of meta-analyses. Neuropsychiatr Dis Treat. 2018;14:165–78. Published 2018 Jan 4. doi: 10.2147/NDT.S138430

38. Dawson KS, Bryant RA, Harper M, et al. Problem management plus (PM+): a WHO transdiagnostic psychological intervention for common mental health problems. World Psychiatry. 2015;14(3):354–57. doi: 10.1002/wps.20255

39. Nakao M, Shirotsuki K, Sugaya N. Cognitive-behavioural therapy for management of mental health and stress-related disorders: recent advances in techniques and technologies. Biopsychosoc Med. 2021;15(1):16. Published 2021 Oct 3. doi: 10.1186/s13030-021-00219-w

12.3 USE OF PHARMACEUTICAL INTERVENTIONS FOR PRIMARY CARE MANAGEMENT OF DEPRESSION AND ANXIETY

Allen F. Shaughnessy and Lisa Cosgrove

DEPRESSION
History of treatment

From 'melancholia' to 'hypochondriasis' to 'the blues' of the past to the 'endogenous depression' of today, healers over time have searched for ways to treat the spectrum of hopelessness, sorrow, dejection, despondency, emptiness, despair and discouragement that, when they persist, lead to a loss of functioning of the individual. From Hippocrates to current guideline writers, authorities have offered options for treatment. Humoral therapy, which governed medical thinking for 2,000 years until the middle of the 19th century, resulted in purgatives prescribed to rid the depressed patient of excess black bile (*melaina chole*). Later, the potent (and quite toxic) stimulant qualities of strychnine in the *Nux vomica* seed led to its use for depressed mood. Electricity, in the form of electroconvulsive therapy, became popular upon its discovery and is still used today.

In a sense, 'rocket science'[1] is responsible for the explosion of drug therapy for depression. At the end of World War II, troops discovered large stockpiles of hydrazine, a rocket fuel used to power German V2 rockets that bombarded England. Caustic and poisonous (and also highly explosive), it was also an inexpensive and simple substrate for pharmaceutical chemists to develop potential drugs. Simple manipulations led to the development of the antitubercular drugs isoniazid and iproniazid, which were found to produce euphoria and even hypomania. The finding that isoniazid inhibits *dia*mine oxidase in *Mycobacterium* led to development of the monoamine hypothesis and the use of monoamine oxidase inhibitors (MAOIs) in depression treatment.

Tricyclic antidepressants were developed through manipulation of the basic chemical structure of antihistamines. Imipramine was initially developed as an antipsychotic; both the antipsychotic chlorpromazine and imipramine were developed from the antihistamine promethazine.[2]

Similarly, fluoxetine, the first selective serotonin uptake inhibitor (SSRI), was explored as a new treatment approach to hypertension and, later, obesity. It was ineffective for either use, but improved mood in subjects led to its exploration for the treatment of depression.[3] The initial success in affecting the symptoms of some patients led to the current 'serotonin deficiency' theory of depression.

The primacy of drug treatment for depression was fostered by the release of the *Diagnostic and Statistical Manual of Mental Disorders, Third Edition* in 1980. This edition of diagnostic criteria introduced the current era of biologic psychiatry, whereby social and psychological explanations of depressive symptoms were subordinated to explanations of 'chemical imbalance' in the brain.

Today, antidepressants are characterised by their putative action on one or two neurotransmitters, mainly norepinephrine, serotonin and dopamine. However, these mechanisms are unlikely to be correct explanations. Fluoxetine affects dopamine and norepinephrine uptake to a greater degree than serotonin as well as binding to serotonin, muscarinic, alpha-1 adrenergic and histamine receptors.[4] Aripiprazole, marketed as a treatment addition to another antidepressant, similarly is non-selective in its effect on neurotransmitters. Recent research has found little difference in serotonin activity between depressed and nondepressed people and no effect of SSRIs on serotonin in the brain.[5]

Evidence of benefit

It is a mistake, though, to think that antidepressants do not work in patients with mild to moderate depression. Approximately 50% of patients will respond to the first medication tried. However, almost the same percentage of patients receiving placebo will have a decrease in symptoms of depression over the same period. No matter what type of antidepressant is studied, response rates between active and placebo treatments will be similar.

In a meta-analysis in 2008 of data submitted to the Food and Drug Administration, including research results not published, the weighted mean improvement was 9.60 points on the Hamilton Rating Scale of Depression (HRSD) in the drug groups and 7.80 in the placebo groups, yielding a mean drug–placebo difference of 1.80 on HRSD improvement scores.[6] A second meta-analysis found 'minimal or non-existent' differences between active and placebo treatments in patients with mild to moderate symptoms.[7]

A network meta-analysis was also published evaluating the effectiveness of 21 antidepressants, finding a 'modest' benefit to treatment in comparison with placebo. Based on analysis of all trial data, it appears that about 15% of patients receiving any antidepressant will have a response clinically greater than if they were to receive placebo.[8]

In addition, the effectiveness of antidepressants to maintain remission of depression symptoms is likely overestimated. While epidemiologic data suggest long-term treatment (9–12 months) reduces the risk of a return of symptoms, there are no long-term studies evaluating the comparative effectiveness of antidepressants with placebo.

This difficulty in showing a difference between active treatment and placebo could be due to several causes, including an expectation effect, conditioning, the natural history of depression or regression to the mean. Placebo treatment, even open-label placebo, in which the patient is told they are being given a placebo, has been shown to be effective to treat pain. In an open-label study to examine the effect of conditioning, 51 patients who had undergone spinal surgery were randomised to receive placebo three times daily in addition to an opioid analgesic taken every four hours as needed. Patients receiving placebo were told that it was inactive but that it should be taken regardless of whether they needed the opioid analgesic. Over the course of the follow-up, patients taking placebo took 30% less opioid analgesic.[9]

It may also be that a substantial proportion of patients wait to seek care for depression symptoms until late in the natural course of the syndrome. Without antidepressant therapy, episodes of clinical depression last from two months to several years, with an average of around five to six months. One-third of the patients recover within a year.

Regression to the mean, another explanation, is a statistical phenomenon in which extreme results measured over time tend to return to average. Tall people tend to have offspring that are not as tall, which is why the human species has only slightly increased in height over the past millennia.

The benefit of treatment, especially when combined with psychotherapy, is more demonstrable in patients with severe depression. For many mental health conditions, psychotherapies (e.g., cognitive behavioural, relational, dialectical behaviour therapy) are established treatment options, with evidence showing that they are as effective as psychotropic medications, and certainly pose less risk.[10] For example, there is strong evidence that psychotherapy is effective in achieving a sustained response as an initial treatment of depression.[11]

Evidence of harm with antidepressants

The question, one with which primary care physicians are quite familiar, 'do antidepressants work?' is, at best, an incomplete one. First, the question of effectiveness is a complicated one. As noted in the previous section, if one relies on clinical trial data that focuses predominantly on the reduction of symptoms as measured by depression scales, the statistical difference found between drug and placebo (typically for more severe depression) may not translate into clinically meaningful change. Additionally, the question of effectiveness must always be weighed against the potential for harm. In this section we address the controversies around antidepressants being linked to increased risk of suicidality and violence, increasing concern about withdrawal symptoms and harms associated with long-term use.

In 2003 the Medicines and Healthcare Products Regulatory Agency (MHRA) recommended that SSRIs should not be used to treat adolescents with major depressive disorders (fluoxetine being the exception). The following year, after an independent review of placebo-controlled trials, the US Food and Drug Administration (FDA) issued a black box warning for nine antidepressants for children and adolescents. In 2007 the FDA expanded their black box warning – the most stringent the regulatory body invokes – to include 18- to 24-year-olds. Although more recent studies, including meta-analyses,[12] observational studies[13] and critical reviews,[14] also concluded that antidepressants may increase the suicide risk in youth, the black box warning has generated controversy and confusion because depression also increases the risk of suicidality. Most researchers and clinicians now agree that antidepressants should be used with great caution in youth and only for severe cases and/or when other interventions have failed. This view is strongly supported by the fact that there is a documented under-reporting of harms in industry-funded clinical trials, particularly for antidepressants and antipsychotics.

For example, in 2015 Le Noury and colleagues conducted a re-analysis of SmithKline Beecham's Study 329, an influential study concluding that paroxetine was safe and effective in adolescents.[15] After obtaining access to the full unpublished dataset, Le Noury et al. found an increase in harms for paroxetine that was not reported in the published literature. Specifically, the researchers concluded that

> Neither paroxetine nor high dose imipramine showed efficacy for major depression in adolescents, and there was an increase in harms with both drugs . . . including suicidal ideation and behaviour and other serious adverse events in the paroxetine group and cardiovascular problems in the imipramine group. . . . Access to primary data from trials has important implications for both clinical practice and research, including that published conclusions about efficacy and safety should not be read as authoritative.

Similarly, a systematic review of randomised controlled trial (RCT) data found that antidepressants "double the occurrence of events that the FDA has defined as possible precursors to suicide and violence".[16] While the issue of causality cannot be determined, there is research that suggests a possible association between SSRIs and convictions for violent crimes for adolescents and young adults (ages 15–24).

There is burgeoning evidence that a discontinuation syndrome occurs in the majority of people who take SSRIs and that this risk is increased if the medication is stopped abruptly, if the SSRI has a shorter half-life and if the treatment duration is long. Common withdrawal symptoms include flu-like symptoms, gastrointestinal problems, sleep disturbances, dizziness, anxiety and sensory disturbances (e.g., some individuals report feeling a sensation of electric shocks or 'brain zaps'). The cause is not known, although it has been suggested that downregulation may play a central role. Unfortunately, while tapering is recommended to prevent or mitigate a discontinuation syndrome, there is limited research and guidance on how to taper or discontinue any psychotropic medications, including antidepressants. It is also important to note that these withdrawal-like symptoms can often be mistaken as the beginning of relapse of the original episode of depression,[17] and thus one should be cautious about immediately reinstating the antidepressant. A slower taper, increased psychosocial supports and psychotherapy, if needed, are the most judicious responses when there is an increase in symptoms. Preliminary discussions about the length of antidepressant treatment should be initiated at the time of prescription, as patients tend to believe it is their physician's responsibility to initiate discussions about discontinuation. Indeed, to enhance the informed consent process, clinicians and patients should, at the outset, collaboratively identify target symptoms, look carefully at the context in which symptoms are manifest, identify any health-harming legal needs (e.g., unsafe or precarious living conditions, discrimination or harassment at work) and discuss a possible duration of treatment and a discontinuation plan at the outset.[18,19]

Cardiovascular effects are most prominent and likely with MAOIs, including the well-known hypertensive crisis that can occur with ingestion of tyramine-containing foods such as aged cheese. Hypotension can also occur. Phenelzine may cause acute myocarditis at high doses, and moclobemide, in overdose, can cause QTc prolongation with resulting arrhythmia.[20]

Tricyclic antidepressants can slow cardiac conduction velocity, especially in people with an underlying conduction defect. They may also cause hypotension or orthostatic hypotension and sinus tachycardia and should be avoided or closely monitored in patients with pre-existing cardiovascular disease.

SSRIs are usually free of cardiac effects, though arrhythmias have been reported. Blood pressure should be monitored in patients receiving venlafaxine and other serotonin and norepinephrine reuptake inhibitors (SNRIs).

Sexual dysfunction has been associated with antidepressant use. The risk seems to be lower with bupropion and may be higher with escitalopram and paroxetine.[21] Falls and fractures, unrelated to postural hypotension, have been associated with SSRI use, especially in the first six weeks of treatment.[22] Hyponatremia is unusual but can occur in older patients already at risk. Gastrointestinal bleeding, especially when used in combination with nonsteroidal anti-inflammatory drugs, can occur with SSRIs. Agomelatine, an atypical antidepressant, can increase liver enzymes, and patients receiving it should have regular liver function testing.

Examples of guidelines around the world

Clinical practice guidelines around the world are similar in their approach, matching therapeutic interventions to the acute severity of symptoms and patient history of previous episodes and responses to treatment. They vary in their emphasis on lifestyle changes and their preference for pharmacotherapy, psychotherapy or both. There is a general move away from treating low-level symptoms with drug therapy.

However, the American Psychiatric Association, which has not updated their recommendations since 2010, recommends drug therapy, psychotherapy, their combination and even electroconvulsive therapy for patients with mild depression. Conversely, the recent United Kingdom National Institute for Health and Care Excellence (NICE) guidelines for treatment of less severe depression (Patient Health Questionnaire [PHQ]-9 score of less than 16) begin with a discussion with the patient of whether they wish to start treatment; if they do, the guidelines suggest exploring a wide range of non-pharmacologic approaches, including individual and group psychotherapy, before considering pharmacologic treatment.[23] Similarly, the Royal Australian and New Zealand College of Psychiatrists recommend lifestyle changes and psychological interventions before starting drug therapy.[24] Malaysian guidelines suggest psychotherapeutic approaches for patients with mild to moderate depression, offering drug therapy to patients who have a history of moderate to severe depression, those who have previously responded to drug therapy, those have not responded to non-drug therapy or those who prefer medication.[25]

The American College of Physicians recommends cognitive behavioural therapy for mild depression, either cognitive behavioural therapy or drug therapy for mild to moderate depression and the combination of both for patients with moderate to severe symptoms.[26]

ANXIETY
History of treatment

Anxiety has been treated for millennia. Alcohol is arguably the longest-used anxiolytic in history. The pharmacological era of treatment began with the discovery and development of barbiturates in the early 1900s. Dependence and toxicity in overdose of barbiturates led to a search for safer treatments. In the early 1950s meprobamate, a so-called minor tranquilliser, was developed as a safer alternative and led to widespread recognition and treatment of anxiety but also in recreational use; just as various substances are group-ingested at 'raves' today, meprobamate would be distributed at social gatherings in the mid-20th century.[3] Greater societal acceptance of the treatment of anxiety-producing life events (think 'mother's little helper') expanded the market, leading to the development by a company in Switzerland of chlordiazepoxide, the first of many benzodiazepines (this company, Roche, would go on to be the world's largest privately owned pharmaceutical company).[27,28]

Buspirone was developed as the first anxiolytic to improve symptoms without causing sedation. SSRIs, originally explored to treat hypertension, were found to have an antidepressant effect and, later, an anxiolytic effect without causing ongoing sedation. Given their effectiveness as compared with placebo and their broad therapeutic index, they have risen to become the first-line pharmacological treatment.

Evidence supporting use

Benzodiazepines are effective for the treatment of anxiety symptoms, rapidly reducing symptoms in both adults and older adults. They are highly tolerated in the short term. However, their use is not recommended by most guidelines, given their association with withdrawal, rebound anxiety and dependence. If used, they should be limited to short-term use for acute anxiety crises. There are many available options that vary in their onset of action and duration.

SSRIs and SNRIs are recommended by most practice guidelines as first-line therapy for generalised anxiety disorder, mainly because of their perceived safety and tolerability as compared with the benzodiazepines. There has been limited research comparing benzodiazepines and second-generation antidepressants. In comparison with diazepam, venlafaxine produced similar response rates but was discontinued more often in one study due to side effects and was less effective in reducing somatic symptoms in the other.[29] In comparison with placebo, they are effective in both younger and older adults. Duloxetine, venlafaxine and escitalopram have the largest amount of trial data showing effectiveness, though fluoxetine, sertraline and mirtazapine also are effective, based on smaller studies. Paroxetine is less well tolerated than other options. SSRIs and SNRIs should be taken regularly to be effective for anxiolysis, with the onset of action of several weeks. Treatment can be continued long-term to maintain control of symptoms.

Both benzodiazepines and second-generation antidepressants are associated with withdrawal symptoms. Discontinuing treatment should occur over several weeks to months with slowly decreased doses to prevent symptoms. Recurrence of anxiety may occur with discontinuation of treatment.

Buspirone is unique among antidepressants in that it reduces anxiety without causing sedation or functional impairment. Its mechanism of action is unknown. In clinical trials it is more effective than placebo and reduces symptoms similar to the benzodiazepine oxazepam and the SSRI sertraline.[30]

It may not be as effective in patients who have previously taken benzodiazepines and who are anticipating an immediate effect.[31] Long-term treatment also does not result in abuse or physical dependence. Its onset of action can be as long as several weeks, so it is not an option for quick resolution of symptoms. It can cause dizziness or drowsiness at the onset of treatment, and it should be initiated at low doses, increasing the dose every three to five days until the maintenance dose is reached. Its effectiveness has not been studied beyond four weeks of treatment, though long-term use is not associated with untoward effects. Some patients (1–2%) will exhibit dizziness or other central nervous system effects upon discontinuation, although gradual discontinuation is not recommended for most patients.

Beta-blockers, which act to suppress the physical effects of anxiety such as shakiness, sweating and racing heart, have been used to treat performance anxiety. However, they do not affect the mental aspects of anxiety such as excessive worry, etc., and are therefore limited to occasional use to suppress outward signs of anxiety.

Sedating antihistamines such as diphenhydramine or hydroxyzine will cause sedation and relieve symptoms of generalised anxiety disorder (GAD).[32] In low-quality studies, hydroxyzine produces equivalent symptom reduction as a benzodiazepine or buspirone. It produced higher levels of drowsiness and sleepiness, though overall acceptability (continuing treatment) and tolerance (overall side effects) were similar.

Ashwagandha (*Withania somnifera*) is an Ayurvedic herb that has been used in India for centuries as a broad-spectrum remedy for many illnesses. It has been formally studied for the treatment of anxiety, showing benefit in two studies but not in a third. The appropriate dose and preparation are not defined, and patients can try different doses and products to determine whether it is effective for them.[33]

Kava (*Piper methysticum*) is made from the roots of the plant. It originates in the islands in the Pacific Ocean, where it is used in social gatherings (its name translates to 'intoxicating pepper'). In four randomised trials, results were heterogeneous, but there may be a modest benefit to treatment. Kava has been associated with rare hepatotoxicity, and some patients will experience headaches.[34]

Lavender oil has been used via inhalation, massage and orally to treat anxiety. Based on low-quality evidence, there is some evidence of benefit with inhalation and massage, with better evidence associated with oral use (80 mg daily).[34]

Examples of guidelines around the world

Treatment with an SSRI is suggested as first-line by most guidelines. However, because there are no trials comparing the long-term outcome of antidepressants with a combination of placebo and psychological treatments, an increasing number of researchers and clinicians are advocating for psychological interventions as a universal first-line treatment step.[35] NICE recommends starting with an SSRI if initial intervention with behavioural change is not effective and psychotherapy is not available or desired.[36] Benzodiazepines are recommended only for short-term use during acute crises. The Royal Australian and New Zealand guidelines also recommend SSRIs based on their effectiveness, overall safety and low misuse potential.[37] The World Federation of Biological Psychiatry also recommends SSRIs, along with SNRIs and pregabalin, as first-line therapy. Other options include buspirone and hydroxyzine, reserving long-term treatment with a benzodiazepine only when other drugs or CBT have failed.[38]

REFERENCES

1. Sandler M. Monoamine oxidase inhibitors in depression: history and mythology. J Psychopharmacol. 1990;4:136–9. doi: 10.1177/026988119000400307
2. Hillhouse TM, Porter JH. A brief history of the development of antidepressant drugs: from monoamines to glutamate. Exp Clin Psychopharmacol. 2015;23:1–21. doi: 10.1037/a0038550
3. DeGrandpre R. The cult of pharmacology: how America became the world's most troubled drug culture. Durham, NC: Duke University Press; 2006.
4. Stegenga J. Medical Nihilism. Oxford University Press; 2018. doi: 10.1093/oso/9780198747048.001.0001
5. Moncrieff J, Cooper RE, Stockmann T, et al. The serotonin theory of depression: a systematic umbrella review of the evidence. Mol Psychiatry. Published Online First: July 20 2022. doi: 10.1038/s41380-022-01661-0
6. Kirsch I, Deacon BJ, Huedo-Medina TB, et al. Initial severity and antidepressant benefits: a meta-analysis of data submitted to the food and drug administration. PLoS Med. 2008;5:e45. doi: 10.1371/journal.pmed.0050045
7. Fournier JC, DeRubeis RJ, Hollon SD, et al. Antidepressant drug effects and depression severity: a patient-level meta-analysis. JAMA. 2010;303:47–53. doi: 10.1001/jama.2009.1943
8. Stone MB, Yaseen ZS, Miller BJ, et al. Response to acute monotherapy for major depressive disorder in randomized, placebo controlled trials submitted to the US food and drug administration: individual participant data analysis. BMJ. 2022;e067606. doi: 10.1136/bmj-2021-067606
9. Flowers KM, Patton ME, Hruschak VJ, et al. Conditioned open-label placebo for opioid reduction after spine surgery: a randomized controlled trial. Pain. 2021;162:1828–39. doi: 10.1097/j.pain.0000000000002185
10. Leichsenring F, Steinert C, Rabung S, et al. The efficacy of psychotherapies and pharmacotherapies for mental disorders in adults: an umbrella review and meta-analytic evaluation of recent meta-analyses. World Psychiatry. 2022;21:133–45. doi: 10.1002/wps.20941
11. Furukawa TA, Shinohara K, Sahker E, et al. Initial treatment choices to achieve sustained response in major depression: a systematic review and network meta-analysis. World Psychiatry. 2021;20:387–96. doi: 10.1002/wps.20906
12. Sharma T, Guski LS, Freund N, et al. Suicidality and aggression during antidepressant treatment: systematic review and meta-analyses based on clinical study reports. BMJ. 2016;352:i65. doi: 10.1136/bmj.i65

13. Barbui C, Esposito E, Cipriani A. Selective serotonin reuptake inhibitors and risk of suicide: a systematic review of observational studies. CMAJ Can Med Assoc J J Assoc Medicale Can. 2009;180:291–7. doi: 10.1503/cmaj.081514

14. Spielmans GI, Spence-Sing T, Parry P. Duty to warn: antidepressant black box suicidality warning is empirically justified. Front Psychiatry. 2020;11:18. doi: 10.3389/fpsyt.2020.00018

15. Le Noury J, Nardo JM, Healy D, et al. Restoring study 329: efficacy and harms of paroxetine and imipramine in treatment of major depression in adolescence. BMJ. 2015;351:h4320. doi: 10.1136/bmj.h4320

16. Molero Y, Lichtenstein P, Zetterqvist J, et al. Selective serotonin reuptake inhibitors and violent crime: a cohort study. PLoS Med. 2015;12:e1001875. doi: 10.1371/journal.pmed.1001875

17. Récalt AM, Cohen D. Withdrawal confounding in randomized controlled trials of antipsychotic, antidepressant, and stimulant drugs, 2000–2017. Psychother Psychosom. 2019;88:105–13. doi: 10.1159/000496734

18. Steingard S. Clinical implications of the drug-centered approach. In: Steingard S, ed. Critical psychiatry: controversies and clinical implications. Cham: Springer International Publishing 2019. 113–35. doi: 10.1007/978-3-030-02732-2_5

19. Bye A. Psychiatrists' accounts of helping patients discontinue antidepressant medication. A discourse analysis. PhD thesis, University of Massachusetts Boston, 2020.

20. Yekehtaz H, Farokhnia M, Akhondzadeh S. Cardiovascular considerations in antidepressant therapy: an evidence-based review. J Tehran Heart Cent. 2013;8:169–76.

21. Reichenpfader U, Gartlehner G, Morgan LC, et al. Sexual dysfunction associated with second-generation antidepressants in patients with major depressive disorder: results from a systematic review with network meta-analysis. Drug Saf. 2014;37:19–31. doi: 10.1007/s40264-013-0129-4

22. Kennedy SH, Lam RW, McIntyre RS, et al. Canadian Network for mood and anxiety treatments (CANMAT) 2016 clinical guidelines for the management of adults with major depressive disorder: section 3. Pharmacological treatments. Can J Psychiatry Rev Can Psychiatr. 2016;61:540–60. doi: 10.1177/0706743716659417

23. Overview | Depression in adults: treatment and management | Guidance | NICE. 2022. https://www.nice.org.uk/guidance/ng222 (accessed Feb 2, 2023).

24. Malhi GS, Bell E, Singh AB, et al. The 2020 royal Australian and new zealand college of psychiatrists clinical practice guidelines for mood disorders: major depression summary. Bipolar Disord. 2020;22:788–804. doi: 10.1111/bdi.13035

25. Malaysian Health Technology Assessment Section (MaHTAS). Management of Depressive Disorder (second edition). https://www.moh.gov.my/moh/resources/Penerbitan/CPG/1)_CPG_Management_Major_Depressive_Disorder_(Second_Edition).pdf (accessed Feb 1, 2023).

26. Qaseem A, Owens DK, Etxeandia-Ikobaltzeta I, et al. Nonpharmacologic and pharmacologic treatments of adults in the acute phase of major depressive disorder: a living clinical guideline from the American college of physicians. Ann Intern Med. Published Online First. January 24 2023. doi: 10.7326/M22-2056

27. Donaldson M, Gizzarelli G, Chanpong B. Oral Sedation: a primer on anxiolysis for the adult patient. Anesth Prog. 2007;54:118–29. doi: 10.2344/0003-3006(2007)54[118:OSAPOA]2.0.CO;2

28. Tone A. Listening to the past: history, psychiatry, and anxiety. Can J Psychiatry Rev Can Psychiatr. 2005;50:373–80. doi: 10.1177/070674370505000702

29. Offidani E, Guidi J, Tomba E, et al. Efficacy and tolerability of benzodiazepines versus antidepressants in anxiety disorders: a systematic review and meta-analysis. Psychother Psychosom. 2013;82:355–62. doi: 10.1159/000353198

30. Treating GAD: Is Buspirone a Good Option? Medscape. https://www.medscape.com/viewarticle/828221 (accessed Feb 2, 2023).
31. DeMartinis N, Rynn M, Rickels K, et al. Prior benzodiazepine use and buspirone response in the treatment of generalized anxiety disorder. J Clin Psychiatry 2000;61: 91–4. doi: 10.4088/jcp.v61n0203
32. Guaiana G, Barbui C, Cipriani A. Hydroxyzine for generalised anxiety disorder. Cochrane Database Syst Rev. 2010;CD006815. doi: 10.1002/14651858.CD006815.pub2
33. Pratte MA, Nanavati KB, Young V, et al. An alternative treatment for anxiety: a systematic review of human trial results reported for the ayurvedic herb ashwagandha (*Withania somnifera*). J Altern Complement Med. 2014;20:901–8. doi: 10.1089/acm.2014.0177
34. DeGeorge KC, Grover M, Streeter GS. Generalized anxiety disorder and panic disorder in adults. Am Fam Physician. 2022;106:157–64.
35. Ormel J, Spinhoven P, de Vries YA, et al. The antidepressant standoff: why it continues and how to resolve it. Psychol Med. 2020;50:177–86. doi: 10.1017/S0033291719003295
36. Generalised Anxiety Disorder and Panic Disorder in Adults: Management. 2020.
37. Andrews G, Bell C, Boyce P, et al. Royal Australian and new zealand college of psychiatrists clinical practice guidelines for the treatment of panic disorder, social anxiety disorder and generalised anxiety disorder. Aust N Z J Psychiatry. 2018;52: 1109–72. doi: 10.1177/0004867418799453
38. Bandelow B, Sher L, Bunevicius R, et al. Guidelines for the pharmacological treatment of anxiety disorders, obsessive-compulsive disorder and posttraumatic stress disorder in primary care. Int J Psychiatry Clin Pract. 2012;16:77–84. doi: 10.3109/13651501.2012.667114

CHAPTER 13

Improving practice

DOI: 10.1201/9781003391531-13

13.1 NICE GUIDELINES ON DEPRESSION AND ANXIETY

Sherina Mohd Sidik and Felicity Goodyear-Smith

The National Institute for Health and Care Excellence (NICE) guidelines are evidence-based recommendations for health and care in England. These guidelines set out the care and services suitable for most people with a specific condition or need and in certain circumstances or settings. The aim is to help health and social care professionals in preventing ill health, promoting and protecting good health, improving the quality of care and services and adapting and providing health and social care services.[1] In this chapter we summarise the recommendations for NICE guidelines for depression and anxiety relevant to primary care.

NICE GUIDELINE ON DEPRESSION

The NICE Guideline on Depression in Adults: Treatment and Management published in 2022 covers identifying, treating and managing depression in people aged 18 years old and above.[2] It is a detailed and comprehensive guide on treatment and management of depression in adults. It recommends treatments for first episodes of depression and further-line treatments and provides advice on preventing relapse and managing chronic depression, psychotic depression and depression with a coexisting diagnosis of personality disorder. Our focus in this brief summary is on the primary care detection and management of depression in adults.

Under principles of care, the guidelines recommend building a trusting relationship and working in an open, engaging and non-judgemental manner with people with depression and their families or carers. Providers should explore the treatment choices in an atmosphere of hope and optimism, explaining the different courses of depression and that recovery is possible. They should be aware that stigma and discrimination can be associated with a diagnosis of depression and that the symptoms of depression itself, and the impact of stigma and discrimination, can make it difficult for people to access mental health services or take up offers of treatment. Steps should be taken to reduce stigma, discrimination and barriers for those seeking help for depression, and discussions should take place in settings where confidentiality, privacy and dignity are respected.

In the section on recognition and assessment, providers are advised to be alert to possible depression, particularly in people with a past history of depression or a chronic physical health problem with associated functional impairment, and to consider asking the two questions (similar to the Patient

Health Questionnaire [PHQ]-2, but over the past month rather than two weeks, with a binary option of yes or no):

1. During the last month, have you often been bothered by feeling down, depressed or hopeless?
2. During the last month, have you often been bothered by having little interest or pleasure in doing things?

If the answer to either question is yes, then a primary care provider should perform a mental health assessment (unless they are not competent to do this, in which case they should refer to someone who can). The assessment should include not just the symptoms but also their severity, duration and previous history of depression, coexisting conditions, current lifestyle and living conditions, any issues with interpersonal relationships and past or recent stressful or traumatic events. People with depression should always be asked about self-harm, suicidal ideation and intent and, where there is risk of this, ensure that appropriate help is available.

There is considerable guidance provided on choice, including shared decision-making, different treatment options (such as psychological and psychosocial interventions and pharmacological treatments), monitoring and preventing relapse. While these guidelines are for health care providers in England, the recommendations are evidence-based, and many are relevant to the detection and management of depression in primary care in other countries.

NICE GUIDELINE FOR ANXIETY

The NICE Guideline on Generalised Anxiety Disorder and Panic Disorder in Adults: Management (www.nice.org.uk/guidance/cg113) was published in 2011 and updated in 2020.[3] It covers the care and treatment of adults (aged 18 and over) with generalised anxiety disorder (GAD), as well as panic disorder.

The principles of care are similar to those when working with people with depression: Build a relationship and work in an open, engaging and non-judgemental manner; explore the person's worries in order to jointly understand the impact of GAD; explore treatment options collaboratively with them, indicating that decision-making is a shared process; and ensure that the discussion takes place in settings in which confidentiality, privacy and dignity are respected.

The provider should be alert to possible anxiety disorders, particularly in people with a past history, possible relevant somatic symptoms or in those who have experienced a recent traumatic event. They should consider initial assessment using the questions from the GAD-2,[4] which asks how often

(4-point Likert scale, from not at all to nearly every day), over the previous two weeks, the person has been bothered by feeling nervous, anxious or on edge and how often they have not been able to stop or control worrying. If the score is 3 or more, a further assessment should be undertaken.

A stepped-care approach is recommended depending on severity, including psychoeducation, options for treatment including psychological and pharmacological interventions (first-line is a selective serotonin reuptake inhibitor [SSRI]) and active monitoring.

These guidelines are produced for English health professionals, but, as mentioned, are likely to also be used in the detection and management of anxiety in primary care in other countries. Note that in Chapter 1 Richard Byng predicts that services in England will move away from the traditional 'diagnose and treat' model of care towards more general support of mental and social well-being, avoiding the medicalisation that comes with diagnostic labels.

REFERENCES

1. NICE Guidelines. Available from: https://www.nice.org.uk/About/What-we-do/Our-Programmes/NICE-guidance/NICE-guidelines (accessed February 22, 2023).
2. NICE Guideline. Depression in adults: treatment and management. Published June 29 2022. www.nice.org.uk/guidance/ng222 (accessed February 22, 2023).
3. NICE Guideline: Generalised anxiety disorder and panic disorder in adults: management. Published January 26 2011. Updated June 15 2020. Available from: www.nice.org.uk/guidance/cg113 (accessed February 22, 2023).
4. Skapinakis P. The 2-item generalized anxiety disorder scale had high sensitivity and specificity for detecting GAD in primary care. Evidence Based Med. 2007;12(5):149. doi: 10.1136/ebm.12.5.149

13.2 A TEAM APPROACH TO HEALTH AND WELL-BEING IN PRIMARY CARE – THE AOTEAROA (NEW ZEALAND) EXAMPLE

Felicity Goodyear-Smith

Aotearoa (New Zealand) has a long history of general practitioners providing first-contact primary care in community-based family practices, working alongside practice nurses.[1] Traditionally general practice provided comprehensive ongoing cradle-to-grave care to patients and their families, catering for both their physical and emotional health and well-being. It is recognised that in most consultations there will be both physical and psychological components. Typically general practitioners and practice nurses provide psychoeducation and simple brief psychological interventions, referring on to community-based counsellors or psychologists or to secondary care psychiatric services when relevant and available.

Indigenous Māori and migrant Pacific people's frameworks, increasingly used in New Zealand, reinforce a holistic model of care. The Māori health Te Whare Tapa Whā model[2] and the Pacific health Fonofale framework[3] both use the metaphor of a meeting house. These are dynamic models promoting the holistic nature of health and well-being and the interactive relationship of their components.

In the Māori model, the four house posts or pillars are the physical, mental, spiritual and family components of health and well-being (Figure 13.1).

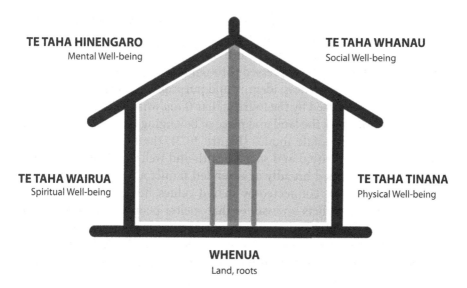

FIGURE 13.1 Te Whare Tapa Whā model.

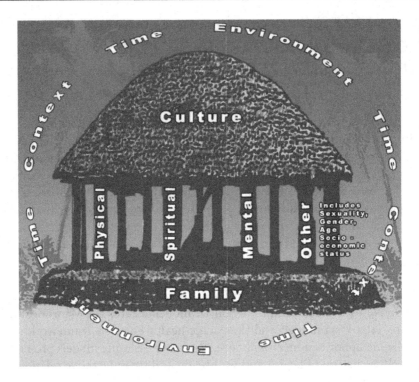

FIGURE 13.2 Fonofale model.

Physical well-being (*taha tinana*) involves taking care of one's body with healthy lifestyle behaviours and managing disease. Mental well-being (*taha hinengaro*) involves emotions, cognition, communication and motivation to achieve goals, not just addressing mental illness or distress. Spiritual well-being (*taha wairua*) may relate to faith or religious beliefs or a connection with the sacred. It may be expressed through beliefs and practices that support a sense of self-awareness, identity and purpose. Family and community well-being is represented by the fourth pillar (*taha whānau*). The foundation of the house (*whare*) is the land and place of belonging (*whenua*).

In the Pacific Fonofale model (Figure 13.2), the four posts (*pou*) are physical, mental, spiritual and social health and well-being, with the family as the floor, defined broadly as extended family and other community member relationships connected by shared values. The roof represents the cultural practices, beliefs and values that shelter people. Surrounding the house (*fale*) is the physical environment, the socio-political context and the point in time. These models also resonate well with the World Health Organization's definition of health as "a state of complete physical, mental and social well-being".[4]

Since 2020 heath improvement practitioners (HIPs) and health coaches have been an emerging workforce within general practice. HIPs are members of the general practice team and are registered health practitioners accredited by Health New Zealand (Te Whatu Ora) to work in the health sector.[5] They have training in providing brief talking therapies and preferably have previously worked in the mental health and addiction field. Any patient who is enrolled in the practice can see a HIP for a 20- to 30-minute consultation either by appointment or in an unbooked session for same-day referrals. Patients do not require any previous or current mental health or addiction diagnosis. When general practice staff see patients whom they identify would benefit from some form of counselling, psychological intervention or other support beyond what they can offer within their 15-minute appointment, they can do a 'warm handover' to an HIP who can see the patient on the same day they are visiting the practice. HIPs can also provide group sessions for a range of issues such as insomnia, gout, anxiety or cardiovascular disease.

Heath coaches are also collaborative members of the general practice team and work closely with HIPs.[6] Their role is to support the practice's enrolled population to address issues that impact on their health and well-being. Health coaching aims to build people's motivation and capability to better understand and self-manage their physical and emotional well-being needs. These may be related to long-term physical or mental health conditions or substance use, but also to everyday emotional or physical well-being challenges. The health coach may use motivational interviewing and other processes that aid behaviour change decisions, and they support patients and their families to access community and online resources which may enhance their social, emotional and physical well-being.

Health coaches are not registered health practitioners but receive training from Te Pou, the national workforce centre of mental health, addiction and disability. Typically health coaches provide support to about 8–10 people a day, including scheduled appointments, warm handovers and meeting with families and groups in practices and other community settings, including homes.

HIPs and health coaches bring value as team players. They have the time and ability to extend the care provided by the primary care practitioners to help patients understand and self-manage their health and well-being needs. The 'corridor' warm handover facilitates further care without the need for formal referral. HIPs and health coaches have a strength-based rather than a deficit-based approach. Diagnostic labels such as depression and anxiety are not required to access their services, and the focus is on supporting cognitive and behavioural changes and self-management. Some early evaluations of HIP training have indicated that trainees highly rate the value of the training programme and demonstrate subsequent increased confidence in their work.[7] However, this is a new initiative. There are no outcome studies to date, although anecdotal evidence suggests that practice staff and patients find the addition of these team members helpful in health care provision in primary care settings.

REFERENCES

1. Goodyear-Smith F, Ashton T. New Zealand health system: universalism struggles with persisting inequities. Lancet. 2019;394(10196):432–42. doi: 10.1016/S0140-6736 (19)31238-3
2. Durie M. Māori health models – Te Whare Tapa Whā Wellington: Ministry of Health. 1984. Available from: https://www.health.govt.nz/our-work/populations/maori-health/ maori-health-models/maori-health-models-te-whare-tapa-wha (accessed April 2021).
3. Pulotu-Endeman F. Fonofale Model of Health. 15. Wellington: (NZ): Mental Health Commission. 2001.
4. World Health Organization. Constitution of the World Health Organization. New York: WHO; 1946:244.
5. Te Pou. Health improvement practitioners in New Zealand Wellington 2023 [cited Jan 2023]. Available from: https://www.tepou.co.nz/initiatives/integrated-primary-mental-health-and-addiction/health-improvement-practitioners-in-new-zealand.
6. Te Pou. Health Coaching Wellington 2023 [cited Jan 2023]. Available from: https://www.tepou.co.nz/initiatives/integrated-primary-mental-health-and-addiction/health-coaching.
7. Te Pou. Health Improvement Practitioner: Training Evaluation Report January to June 2022. Wellington. 2022:22.

13.3 INTEGRATING PHYSICAL AND MENTAL HEALTH SERVICES IN PRIMARY CARE

Mehmet Akman

Mental disorders are prevalent in all societies. In 2019, 418 million disability-adjusted life years (DALYs) could be attributed to mental disorders (16% of global DALYs).[1] In contrast with the high prevalence, the number of people receiving treatment and care among the patients diagnosed with mental disorders is relatively low, yielding a significant treatment gap. Taking into consideration the increased health care accessibility when strong primary care is built into the community, this treatment gap can be decreased when mental and physical health services are integrated within primary care. Mental health problems often coexist with physical health problems, and this coexistence will be more dominant in an ageing population. Integrated primary care services help ensure that people are treated holistically, meeting the mental health needs of people with physical disorders, as well as the physical health needs of people with mental disorders. Primary care services for mental health are less expensive than psychiatric hospitals for patients, communities and governments alike. In addition, patients and families avoid indirect costs associated with seeking specialist care in distant locations.[2] The benefits of integrated models of care include reduced admissions (especially for chronic conditions), reduced mortality and improved overall disease management and have additional benefits in terms of cost-effectiveness of service delivery.[3]

Together with diagnosable mental health problems, subthreshold symptoms are common in primary care and often coexist with high levels of complexity and challenging social circumstances, such as unemployment and poor housing. Medically unexplained symptoms and substance abuse disorders are also highly prevalent in primary care.[4] These problems are often considered minor and poorly managed due to fragmented service provision. Outcomes of physical health problems are worse when comorbid with mental disorders. Several risk factors have been attributed to this association, including reduced adherence to treatment and increased social risk factors among patients with mental disorders, for example, high rates of smoking, lower levels of physical activity and poorer dietary intake. Many studies have recommended targeted screening programmes, particularly in primary care, for those with diagnosed mental disorders to prevent the onset or reduce the progression of comorbid physical conditions.[2]

HOW TO INTEGRATE?

Primary care workers' pre-service and/or in-service training on mental health issues is an essential prerequisite for mental health integration.

Additionally, health workers also must receive specialist supervision over time. Collaborative or shared care models, in which joint consultations and interventions are held between primary care workers and mental health specialists, are an auspicious way of providing ongoing training and support. However, the tasks attributed to primary care must be limited and doable. Only then will primary care workers be able to function well. The functions of primary care workers may be expanded as practitioners gain skills and confidence. The integration process must be accompanied by complementary services, particularly secondary care components to which primary care workers can turn for referrals, support and supervision. This support can come from community mental health centres, secondary-level hospitals or skilled practitioners working specifically within the primary care system. Specialists may range from psychiatric nurses to psychiatrists.

Access to essential psychotropic medications is crucial for holistic and comprehensive care, including mental health problems. This requires the direct distribution of psychotropic medicines to primary care facilities, rather than through psychiatric hospitals. Legislation and regulations must be reviewed and updated to allow primary care workers to prescribe and dispense psychotropic medications, mainly where mental health specialists and physicians are scarce.[2]

Funding is another essential part of the integrated mental and physical health provision at the primary care level. In the case of incentives, precaution is needed for not enhancing selective patient care for mental disorders. Legal/regulatory challenges pertain to the practice of non-physician personnel for prescribing and counselling. Integrated care also requires revising the role of the physician and the distribution of functions among the team.[5]

EXAMPLES IN PRACTICE

In London in the United Kingdom, a 'Primary Care Psychotherapy Consultation Service' was provided by a multidisciplinary team of mental health professionals to help primary care doctors (PCDs) manage complex patients (for example, those with medically unexplained symptoms, comorbidity or personality disorders). This service included direct one-to-one consultations with patients, joint consultations with PCDs and a significant emphasis on training and skills transfer. Outcomes included increased confidence among PCDs, significant improvements in mental health and functioning and reduced service use in primary care.[4]

There are several other examples of collaboration between health professionals to improve primary care services for patients with mental and physical multimorbidity. A randomised controlled study comparing collaborative and usual care at the primary care level in north-west England found that coordinated care that incorporates brief low-intensity psychological therapy delivered in partnership with practice nurses in primary care can reduce depression and improve self-management of chronic disease in people with mental and physical multimorbidity.[5]

In the United States, a randomised trial in Washington state reported that diabetic or cardiac patients with depression benefited from integrated primary care provided in a team-based approach in terms of dietary changes and increased exercise compared to usual care.[6] The Medicaid health home model in the United States is another example of integrating physical and mental health care. Collaborative care programmes are used as an approach for integration in which primary care providers, care managers and psychiatric consultants work together to provide care and monitor patients' progress. These programmes are both clinically and financially effective for various mental health conditions in multiple settings, using several different payment mechanisms. Collaborative care implemented in Medicaid homes includes (1) care coordination and care management, (2) regular/proactive monitoring and treatment to target using validated clinical rating scales and (3) regular consultation for patients who do not show clinical improvement. According to this experience, implementing evidence-based collaborative care could substantially improve medical and mental health outcomes and functioning and reduce health care costs.[7]

A trial was conducted in rural Australia for an integrated model for primary care settings to coordinate mental and physical health care. This is particularly important given that there are very few specialists in rural areas. The rural Australian experience showed that integrated physical and mental health service models that focus on building local service provider relationships and are responsive to community needs and outcomes seem to be more beneficial in rural settings than top-down approaches that focus on policies, formal structures and governance.[8] To maximise service effectiveness for people with severe and persistent mental illness, approaches that concentrate on integration around the patient pathway and frontline team should be emphasised. Such an approach designed within local resource capacity limits is more likely to maximise practitioner knowledge and involvement and be financially and clinically sustainable.

In a recent scoping review exploring models of integration for mental and physical health, 37 models were identified from the literature.[9] According to the authors, it is evident that models are well received by consumers and providers, increase service access and improve physical and mental health outcomes. Key characteristics of the models include shared information technology, financial integration, a single entry point, co-located care, multidisciplinary teams and meetings, care coordination, joint treatment plans, joint treatment, joint assessment, agreed referral criteria and person-centred care.

A recent qualitative study explored facilitators and barriers to integrating physical and mental health at the primary care level. Integration is facilitated by the co-location of providers within the same department, a warm hand-off, collaborative and collegial relationships, strong leadership support and a shared electronic health record. However, interdisciplinary conflict, power differentials, job insecurity, communication challenges and the subsumption of mental health into the medical model can all pose barriers to successful integration. Interdisciplinary cultural conflict plays an important role, and some mental health providers wanted to engage patients in long-term therapy. In contrast, medical care providers have more control over resource allocation and expected short, effective, efficient interventions. In addition, mental health providers reported concern about the focus being on productivity, emphasising quantity rather than quality of care.[10] To overcome these barriers, clear communication is essential between mental health and primary care workers.

A report from the King's Fund identifies two areas of improvement for general practice: (1) Improving management of medically unexplained symptoms in primary care and (2) strengthening primary care for the physical health needs of people with severe mental illnesses.[11]

CONCLUSION

In conclusion, the evidence we have today favours integration between physical and mental health at the primary care level. However, future research is still needed to identify the priorities of communities and service providers and also to clarify integrated care features associated with positive outcomes at lower costs. To successfully integrate mental and physical health, primary care workers need to be trained appropriately, team-based interprofessional collaboration is essential and a holistic approach that offers reliable symptom control while dealing with other clinical, psychological and social needs is necessary.

REFERENCES

1. Arias D, Saxena S, Verguet S. Quantifying the global burden of mental disorders and their economic value. eClin Med. Sep 28 2022;54:101675.
2. Funk M, Ivbijaro G. Integrating mental health into primary care: a global perspective. World Health Organization and World Organization of Family Doctors (WONCA). WHO Geneva; 2008:206.
3. Fogarty F, McCombe G, Brown K, Van Amelsvoort T, Clarke M, Cullen W. Physical health among patients with common mental health disorders in primary care in Europe: a scoping review. Ir J Psychol Med. 2021;38(1):76–92.
4. Das P, Naylor C, Majeed A. Bringing together physical and mental health within primary care: a new frontier for integrated care. J R Soc Med. 2016;109(10):364–66.
5. Coventry P, Lovell K, Dickens C, Bower P, Chew-Graham C, McElvenny D, Hann M, Cherrington A, Garrett C, Gibbons CJ, Baguley C, Roughley K, Adeyemi I, Reeves D, Waheed W, Gask L. Integrated primary care for patients with mental and physical multimorbidity: cluster randomised controlled trial of collaborative care for patients with depression comorbid with diabetes or cardiovascular disease. BMJ. 2015;350:h638.

6. Rosenberg D, Lin E, Peterson D, Ludman E, Von Korff M, Katon W. Integrated medical care management and behavioral risk factor reduction for multicondition patients: behavioral outcomes of the TEAMcare trial. Gen Hosp Psychiatry. 2014;36(2):129–34. Epub 2013 Nov 4.

7. Unützer J. Collaborative Care Model: An Approach for Integrating Physical and Mental Health Care in Medicaid Health Homes. Center for healthcare strategies. Policy Brief. 2013. Downloaded from www.chcs.org/resource/the-collaborative-care-model-an-approach-for-integrating-physical-and-mental-health-care-in-Medicaid-health-homes/ (accessed January 15, 2023).

8. Fitzpatrick SJ, Perkins D, Handley T, Brown D, Luland T, Corvan E. Coordinating mental and physical health care in rural Australia: an integrated model for primary care settings. Int J Integr Care. 2018;18(2):19.

9. Coates D, Coppleson D, Schmied V. Integrated physical and mental healthcare: an overview of models and their evaluation findings. Int J Evid Based Healthc. 2020;18(1):38–57.

10. Monaghan K, Cos T. Integrating physical and mental healthcare: facilitators and barriers to success. Med Point Care. 2021;5. doi: 10.1177/23992026211050615

11. Naylor C, Das P, Ross S, Honeyman M, Thompson J, Gilburt H. Bringing together physical and mental health. The King's Fund; 2016 https://www.kingsfund.org.uk/publications/physical-and-mental-health/priorities-for-integrating

CHAPTER 14

Conclusion

Sherina Mohd Sidik and Felicity Goodyear-Smith

Our book starts with a global perspective from Dawit Wondimagegn. He explains that depression, anxiety and medically unexplained symptoms are common and present a significant burden to individuals, family and society at large around the world. Despite the availability of appropriate interventions, he expresses concern that their detection, diagnosis and treatment in primary care are limited. He advocates for increased development and implementation of mental health policies and programmes at all levels across the globe.

Richard Bying presents an alternative view, namely that feeling low or anxious is part of the human condition. He argues that rather than defining these problems as disorders or diseases which need detecting and treating, the focus should be on supporting people in their journey through life, struggling to deal with the mainly social challenges they meet.

In Chapter 3, we outline some of the tools used for assessing depression and anxiety in primary care. We discuss whether mass screening is justified under the accepted criteria of screening, as well as the risk of both under- or over-diagnosing and of under- or over-intervening.

There follows 20 case histories from countries across all regions of the world, with high-, middle- and low-income examples. In these descriptions, the authors all present information on the prevalence of depression and anxiety in their country, how these conditions manifest, diagnosis, management, challenges and future directions.

The picture they paint is varied. Prevalence ranges from a low of 4.6% depression and 5.6% anxiety in Ecuador to a high of 11.2% depression and 29% anxiety in Australia. However, it should be noted that the prevalence

DOI: 10.1201/9781003391531-14

figures provided are not necessarily comparable, as some report on national data, some on community-based or primary care data and others on smaller studies. Most authors consider that these conditions are very prevalent in their country, and they consider that identifying cases and making these diagnoses in their patients is helpful.

Screening for these conditions in primary care varies greatly. It is routine in Malaysia; takes place when clinical symptoms indicate in countries such as Ghana, Australia, Luxemburg and Pakistan; but is rarely, if ever, done in Nepal. Our Canadian author expressed caution about routine screening, which is not currently recommended by the Canadian Task Force on Preventive Health Care. South African colleagues were wary about diagnosing depression and anxiety, given the limited availability of treatment in primary care.

Where treatment is indicated, most countries start with psychological therapies and add medications when there is an inadequate response. In a few countries, for example, Argentina, the initial management is pharmacological. In most of the countries, the family doctor is the main point of contact and gatekeeper for patient management. Many countries (for example, Malaysia, Nigeria, Ghana, Australia, Egypt and Luxembourg) provide family doctors with training to detect, manage and monitor patients with mental health problems in primary care.

The next section of our book deals with vulnerable populations. David Ponka addresses common mental health problems in migrants to Canada, including the issue of complex post-traumatic stress disorder. Mehmet Ungan and Aysegul Cömert discuss mental health issues experienced by refugees in Türkiye and the screening programme run there for migrants heading to the United States. The Russian-Ukrainian war is resulting in both internally and externally displaced Ukrainians and refugees, as well as those who remain living in areas affected by the war. Victoria Tkachenko discusses the effects on the mental health of Ukrainians in her war-torn country.

Vinicius Fischer and colleagues cover a range of psychotherapeutic interventions used for depression and anxiety in primary care, and Allen Shaughnessy and Lisa Cosgrove outline various medications used in pharmaceutical management. It is noted that effectiveness is limited and that the numbers needed to treat for psychotherapeutic interventions are often about four or five, meaning that only a minority of patients will benefit. Anna Stavdal extols the benefits of 'watchful waiting', reducing the medicalising of patients' experiences of feeling low or worried into depression and anxiety. She advocates the use of time to distinguish normal reactions to situational crises from mental illness, with patient and clinician watching and waiting together, and seeing if strategies to tackle existential struggles can be employed.

The penultimate chapter looks at ways that practice might be improved. We cover the latest National Institute for Health and Care Excellence (NICE) guidelines on depression and anxiety and the stepped-care management they recommend, from psychoeducation, through to psychological, pharmacological interventions and then referral to secondary specialist services. An example of moving from a general practitioner to a team-based holistic approach to health and well-being in primary care is given from Aotearoa (New Zealand), including the introduction of heath improvement practitioners and health coaches into the primary care workforce. Finally, Mehmet Akman discusses the integration of physical and mental health services in primary care settings.

A core feature of family medicine is the trusted relationship between clinician and patient. Many, or even most, primary care consultations have a mental health element, even if this is just a patient worrying that symptoms have a sinister cause, rather than merely being benign and self-limiting and seeking reassurance. Changes in mood are part of the human condition. We may be elated when things are going well, or down in the dumps when what we hoped for or expected has not gone according to plan. We grieve when a loved one dies, when a marriage breaks down or when we lose a friend. We may worry about many aspects of our lives – our heath, our financial situation, our family or how we are doing at school or at work, or feel anxious when confronted with difficult or complicated situations.

At one end of the spectrum are the ups and downs of everyday life. It is important not to pathologise normal experiences. However, at the other end there is a point at which emotional responses go beyond situational reactions and cause serious dysfunction. When people feel persistently hopeless, worthless and suicidal, they are likely to be suffering from severe depression. When a feeling of dread or fear persists for months with no obvious cause to the extent that it becomes disabling and interferes with daily life functioning, the patient may meet the diagnostic criteria for generalised anxiety disorder. Ongoing, long-lasting painful emotions around loss preventing resumption of normal life may become persistent grief. These are mental health disorders that warrant intervention.

Time is a key tool in family medicine. We can give our patients time, while providing support, to see whether their symptoms progress to those of a diagnostic mental disorder. We do not wish to miss diagnosing a major psychiatric condition amenable to treatment, but we also need to prevent over-diagnosing resolvable normal reactions to stressful events.

People react differently to stressful situations. Some people are more emotionally labile than others, have greater mood swings and may respond in different ways when exposed to traumatic events. Family medicine involves caring for our patients' mental, spiritual and social health and well-being while attending to their physical and medical needs. We can use our compassion and our problem-solving knowledge to help our patients develop resilience – to be better able to work through emotional pain and suffering. We can support and assist them to develop skills to cope with adversity. Primary care can offer coaching to enable people to make healthier lifestyle choices around eating, exercise, use of alcohol or drugs and social relationships.

There will be times when our patients have clear and prolonged symptoms and signs of clinical depression or anxiety requiring intervention, using the stepped-care approach of psychoeducation, psychotherapy, medication or referral to secondary services, and we need to be alert to these possibilities.

Physical and mental health are not separate entities. As general practitioners, we provide holistic care for our patients and their families. Regardless of whether we consider a patient's distress is a normal reaction to challenging or difficult circumstances or we decide that the criteria for depression or anxiety is met, our role is to assist them with their lifestyle choices and help improve their health and well-being.

Index

Note: Locators in *italics* represent figures and **bold** indicate tables in the text.

Printed in the United States
by Baker & Taylor Publisher Services